THE WISDOM DIET

Eating for Cognitive Longevity

Anthony Ryan Crowley

S.D.N Publishing

Copyright © 2023 S.D.N Publishing

All rights reserved

The characters and events portrayed in this book are fictitious. Any similarity to real persons, living or dead, is coincidental and not intended by the author.

No part of this book may be reproduced, or stored in a retrieval system, or transmitted in any form or by any means, electronic, mechanical, photocopying, recording, or otherwise, without express written permission of the publisher.

ISBN: 9798861297622

CONTENTS

Title Page
Copyright
General Disclaimer   1
Chapter 1: A Mindful Approach to Eating and Thinking   3
Chapter 2: The Cortex and the Kitchen: Where Brain Meets Diet   6
Chapter 3: Neuroscience 101: The Basics of Brain Function   9
Chapter 4: Cracking the Code: Decoding Nutritional Labels   12
Chapter 5: The Cognition Menu: Foods that Fuel Your Brain   15
Chapter 6: The Brain's Favorite Spice: How Curcumin Can Help   18
Chapter 7: Sip to Sharpen: The Benefits of Hydration   21
Chapter 8: The Sugar Conundrum: Sweet But Not So Innocent   24
Chapter 9: The Protein Perspective: Building Blocks of the Brain   27
Chapter 10: Vitamin Velocity: Speeding Up Mental Acuity   30
Chapter 11: Minding Your Gut: The Brain-Gut Connection   33
Chapter 12: Portion Control: How Much is Just Right?   36
Chapter 13: Carb-Loaded or Carb-Limited?   39
Chapter 14: Fishy Business: The Role of Omega-3s   42

Chapter 15: Timing is Everything: When to Eat for Cognitive Power	45
Chapter 16: Antioxidant Arsenal: Foods That Fight Cognitive Decline	48
Chapter 17: Mindful Munching: The Practice of Mindful Eating	51
Chapter 18: Move to Think: Exercise as Cognitive Fuel	54
Chapter 19: Caffeine and Cognition: A Love-Hate Relationship	57
Chapter 20: The Mindful Shopper: Grocery Shopping for Brain Health	60
Chapter 21: Caloric Restriction: Less Might Be More	63
Chapter 22: Intermittent Fasting: A Time to Think	66
Chapter 23: The Cheat Day Dilemma: Indulgence and Cognitive Health	69
Chapter 24: Meal Prep Mindset: Planning for Cognitive Success	72
Chapter 25: Cooking for Cognition: Techniques and Recipes	75
Chapter 26: Supplement Savvy: Do You Need Extra Help?	78
Chapter 27: Culinary Cultures: What We Can Learn from Global Diets	81
Chapter 28: Brain-Friendly Booze? The Alcohol Question	84
Chapter 29: Hormones and Health: Eating for Hormonal Balance	87
Chapter 30: Eating Your Emotions: Food and Mood	90
Chapter 31: Breaking Bad Habits: The Path to Better Choices	93
Chapter 32: The Organic Debate: To Go Organic or Not?	96
Chapter 33: Screen Time Snacking: The Impact of Digital Distraction	99
Chapter 34: Eating Through the Ages: Adapting Your Diet	102

as You Age

Chapter 35: Gender Matters: Tailoring Diet for Men and Women — 105

Chapter 36: Mind over Matter: The Power of Positive Thinking — 108

Chapter 37: Family Fare: Cognitive Nutrition for All Ages — 111

Chapter 38: Culinary Creativity: Making Healthy Eating Enjoyable — 114

Chapter 39: Traveler's Mind: Eating Wisely On the Go — 117

Chapter 40: Conclusion: The Road Ahead — 120

THE END — 123

GENERAL DISCLAIMER

This book is intended to provide general information to the reader on the topics covered. The author and publisher have made every effort to ensure that the information herein is accurate and up-to-date at the time of publication. However, they do not warrant or guarantee the accuracy, completeness, adequacy, or currency of the information contained in this book. The author and publisher expressly disclaim any liability or responsibility for any errors or omissions in the content herein.

The information, guidance, advice, tips, and suggestions provided in this book are not intended to replace professional advice or consultation. Readers are strongly encouraged to consult with an appropriate professional for specific advice tailored to their situation before making any decisions or taking any actions based on the content of this book.

The views and opinions expressed in this book are those of the author and do not necessarily reflect the official policy or position of any other agency, organization, employer or company.

The author and publisher are not responsible for any actions taken or not taken by the reader based on the information, advice, or suggestions provided in this book. The reader is solely responsible for their actions and the consequences thereof.

This book is not intended to be a source of legal, business, medical or psychological advice, and readers are cautioned to seek the services of a competent professional in these or other areas of expertise.

All product names, logos, and brands are property of their respective owners. All company, product and service names used in this book are for identification purposes only. Use of these names, logos, and brands does not imply endorsement.

Readers of this book are advised to do their own due diligence when it comes to making decisions and all information, products, services and advice that have been provided should be independently verified by your own qualified professionals.

By reading this book, you agree that the author and publisher are not responsible for your success or failure resulting from any information presented in this book.

CHAPTER 1: A MINDFUL APPROACH TO EATING AND THINKING

Welcome to the beginning of a culinary journey designed to enrich not just your palate, but your mental canvas. Most diets target your waistline; this one aims a bit higher—at your brain. Let's embark on a gastronomic expedition that's focused on cognitive longevity.

Food as Information for the Brain

Imagine your brain as a supercomputer, continuously performing complex operations. The quality of these operations depends on the quality of data you input, and in this analogy, food serves as that data. A potato chip, for instance, carries a different set of "instructions" than a blueberry does for your brain. While the chip may tell your brain to inflame and slow down, the blueberry signals it to enhance memory and protect against cell damage. When you eat, you're not just consuming calories; you're delivering a packet of information that can alter gene expression, hormone levels, and enzymatic reactions, all of which shape your cognitive landscape.

Neuroplasticity and Nutrients

Neuroplasticity is your brain's ability to reorganize itself by forming new neural connections. Think of it as your mind's agility training. This remarkable ability is influenced by various factors including your life experiences, stress levels, and yes, your diet. Foods rich in antioxidants, omega-3 fatty acids, and other essential nutrients serve as the building blocks that help your brain adapt and evolve, even as you age.

Hacking into the Reward System

Modern-day foods often hack into our brain's reward system, tricking us into craving sugar-laden, high-fat options. This might have served us well in a prehistoric setting where high-calorie foods were scarce, but in today's world of abundance, it's a cognitive disaster. Understanding this reward system is crucial, as the foods that hijack this system are also the ones that contribute to cognitive decline.

Creating a Cognitive Pantry

Your kitchen can be either a pharmacy or a fast lane to mental fog. When stocking your pantry, think about adding foods that serve as cognitive enhancers. Opt for fruits and vegetables with vibrant colors, lean proteins, and an array of spices that do more than just add flavor—they enhance brain function. Toss out those highly processed foods; they're like malware for your mind.

Why "The Wisdom Diet"?

So why name this diet focused on cognitive longevity "The Wisdom Diet"? It's simple. Wisdom is the epitome of cognitive growth, a manifestation of accumulated knowledge, rationality, and emotional resilience. It's what we all aspire to as we age. And it's no secret that a sharp, resilient mind forms the cornerstone of wisdom.

In the coming chapters, we will dive deep into the nitty-gritty of how exactly food interacts with your brain, what to eat, what to avoid, and how to make all of this sustainable. We'll explore nutritional labels, the benefits of hydration, the downside of sugar, and even look into some spices that should be a part of every wise person's diet.

So here's to eating wisely and thinking wisely—because as you'll soon discover, the two are more connected than you might have ever imagined.

CHAPTER 2: THE CORTEX AND THE KITCHEN: WHERE BRAIN MEETS DIET

Introduction

You might not see any visible connection between the bustling activities in your kitchen and the complex neural operations in your cortex, the outer layer of your brain responsible for higher cognitive functions. But make no mistake: what happens in one profoundly influences the other. This chapter pulls back the curtain on the intricate relationship between diet and brain health.

The Neurotransmitter Connection

If you think of your brain as a series of electric circuits, neurotransmitters are the electrical signals that flow through those circuits. They're essential for mood regulation, memory, and cognition. Foods rich in amino acids—think turkey, eggs, and nuts—are precursors to neurotransmitters like serotonin and dopamine. In simpler terms, the turkey sandwich you had for lunch might just be the reason behind your upbeat mood and heightened focus. However, amino acids don't work in isolation; they rely on other nutrients like B vitamins and omega-3 fatty acids to produce a balanced neurotransmitter profile. This is why a balanced diet is pivotal for optimal brain function.

The Anti-Inflammatory Influence

Brain inflammation isn't just a byproduct of injury; it can also result from a diet rich in processed foods, sugars, and unhealthy fats. Chronic inflammation has been linked to cognitive decline, memory loss, and even conditions like Alzheimer's. Foods such as berries, turmeric, and fatty fish are potent anti-inflammatory agents that can neutralize this harmful process. They contain compounds like curcumin and anthocyanins that actively work to reduce inflammation, thereby protecting the brain.

Blood Sugar and Brain Fog

The rush from consuming sugary drinks or processed snacks is not merely a figure of speech; it has its roots in neuroscience. High sugar intake spikes blood glucose levels, leading to a sudden surge of energy. But what goes up must come down—this spike is usually followed by a crash that leaves you feeling mentally foggy. Maintaining a stable blood sugar level through a balanced diet rich in complex carbohydrates, protein, and healthy fats can stave off this cognitive roller coaster.

The Fats of the Matter

Fats often get a bad rap, but they're not all villains in the narrative of nutrition. Your brain is predominantly made up of fats, particularly a type called DHA, found in omega-3 fatty acids. While saturated fats found in fast food can contribute to cognitive decline, omega-3s have been shown to enhance memory, improve mental acuity, and even protect against psychiatric disorders. Foods such as walnuts, chia seeds, and salmon are excellent sources of these beneficial fats.

Brain-Gut Dialogue

The gut isn't just responsible for digestion; it also communicates with the brain through a bidirectional relationship commonly known as the gut-brain axis. Gut flora, or the microbiome, can influence mental health. Prebiotics and probiotics found in foods like yogurt, sauerkraut, and whole grains nourish beneficial bacteria in the gut. These bacteria, in turn, produce neurotransmitters and other compounds that signal the brain, affecting mood and cognitive function.

Conclusion

The ties between your cortex and your kitchen are not just casual connections; they are fundamental relationships that shape your mental well-being. By understanding the biochemistry of neurotransmitters, the anti-inflammatory power of certain foods, the risks of high sugar intake, the essential role of fats, and the mysterious brain-gut dialogue, you'll be better equipped to prepare a diet tailored for cognitive longevity. In the grand scheme of things, your kitchen isn't just a room where food is prepared; it's a neurochemical lab that holds the secrets to a sharper, more resilient mind.

CHAPTER 3: NEUROSCIENCE 101: THE BASICS OF BRAIN FUNCTION

Introduction

We've set the stage with the fascinating dance between the brain and diet. Now it's time to delve deeper into the core mechanics of your cerebral hardware. Understanding the essentials of neuroscience isn't just for lab-coated scientists; it's vital for anyone who wants to take proactive steps to enhance their cognitive longevity.

The Brain's Main Regions

Your brain is composed of several key areas, each responsible for different aspects of cognition and function. The main ones are:

- Frontal Lobe: Responsible for complex thought processes, decision-making, and planning.
- Parietal Lobe: Manages spatial orientation and sensory input.
- Temporal Lobe: Involved in memory and auditory processing.
- Occipital Lobe: Processes visual information.

- Cerebellum: Coordinates voluntary movements and balance.

Knowing which region controls what allows us to focus our dietary approaches on particular cognitive skills.

Neurons: The Cellular Units of Thought

Imagine the brain as an intricate communication network. Neurons are the cellular operators facilitating the exchange of messages through electrical impulses. Their action is mediated by neurotransmitters, chemicals that transmit signals between neurons. When you eat food rich in nutrients like Omega-3 fatty acids, you're essentially fortifying these microscopic operators.

Neurotransmitters and Mood

Serotonin, dopamine, and norepinephrine are the 'feel-good' neurotransmitters you may have heard of. They influence mood, focus, and even hunger. Some nutrients, like tryptophan, can help increase the availability of these neurotransmitters, providing a natural mood boost. Inversely, foods high in sugar and saturated fats can create neurotransmitter imbalances, causing mood swings and cognitive sluggishness.

Blood-Brain Barrier: The Brain's Immigration Office

The blood-brain barrier acts as a protective security system, regulating the substances that can enter the brain from the bloodstream. Certain nutrients, like flavonoids found in blueberries, have been found to cross this barrier, thereby enhancing cognitive function. Understanding this can help us strategize how to introduce beneficial nutrients into our diet.

Brain Plasticity: The Never-Ending Evolution

Once thought to be rigid and unchanging, we now know the brain possesses plasticity, meaning it can change and adapt. Diet is one variable that can influence this plasticity. Nutrients like antioxidants can encourage the development of new neurons, even in adulthood, showing that you can teach an old brain new tricks.

Conclusion

Understanding the basics of brain function is essential for anyone aiming to boost cognitive longevity through diet. It provides the necessary context for understanding why certain foods are termed 'brain foods' and others cognitive culprits. Equipped with this knowledge, you are better positioned to make dietary choices that not only satiate your taste buds but also satiate your neurons, supporting your brain's complex and ever-changing needs.

CHAPTER 4: CRACKING THE CODE: DECODING NUTRITIONAL LABELS

Introduction

You're standing in a grocery aisle, bombarded by shelves upon shelves of packaged food options. Your gut says, "Pick the one that looks delicious!" but your brain chimes in with, "Hold on, is it good for me?" Here's where the alchemy of reading nutritional labels comes in handy. Let's dissect the coded language of nutritional facts and learn how to make choices that your brain will thank you for.

The Ubiquitous Nutrition Facts Panel

Don't be fooled by flashy packaging or clever marketing terms like "all-natural" or "brain-boosting." Those may lure you in, but they don't give you the complete story. Your main go-to should be the Nutrition Facts panel, typically located on the back or side of the package. This information haven will list the serving size, calories, and macronutrients (fats, carbohydrates, and protein), among other details. When selecting foods with cognitive benefits, pay special attention to saturated fats, sugars, and sodium—these are often the hidden culprits in otherwise "healthy" foods.

Micronutrients That Matter

Just as important as macronutrients are micronutrients—those tiny elements that often go unnoticed but play a significant role in cognitive function. Key vitamins like B12, folate, and vitamin D can often be found listed under the 'Vitamin and Minerals' section. These are involved in neural development and neurotransmitter signaling. Also, look out for elements like iron, which aids in oxygen transportation to the brain, and zinc, which is involved in nerve signaling.

The Ingredient List Deciphered

It might seem like you need a Ph.D. in linguistics to understand some of the words listed in the ingredients section. However, a good rule of thumb is the simpler, the better. If you find yourself buried in unpronounceable chemicals, you might want to reconsider your choice. Ingredients are listed in descending order by weight, so ensure that the first few ingredients are whole foods like fruits, vegetables, or whole grains. These are likely to contain the phytonutrients and antioxidants that contribute to cognitive longevity.

The Fiber and Sugar Conundrum

Soluble fiber is a nutritional superstar when it comes to supporting brain health. It not only helps regulate blood sugar levels but also aids in lowering cholesterol. Foods rich in fiber, like oats and whole grains, are beneficial in reducing the risk of cognitive decline. On the flip side, be cautious of added sugars. Though sugar might offer a quick energy spike, it often leads to a rapid crash, affecting your focus and memory. Instead, aim for foods that offer natural sweetness from fruits or other natural sources.

The Art of Serving Size and Calories

Don't be misled by seemingly low-calorie counts on the package. Often these are for unrealistically small serving sizes. Remember, overeating, even healthy foods, can lead to caloric surpluses that are detrimental to both your waistline and brain health. Conversely, starving your body of necessary calories can lead to decreased cognitive function. So, always double-check the serving size and adjust your portions accordingly.

Conclusion

Decoding nutritional labels can be likened to acquiring a second language; initially, it seems daunting, but over time, it becomes second nature. And just like learning a new language enriches your life, so does mastering the language of nutritional labels. They become your internal compass, steering you towards foods that not only satisfy your palate but also fortify your cognitive wellbeing. So, the next time you're caught in the whirlwind of choices at your grocery store, you'll know exactly what to look for. Armed with this knowledge, you become the Sherlock Holmes of nutritional sleuthing, always on the case for brain-boosting eats.

CHAPTER 5: THE COGNITION MENU: FOODS THAT FUEL YOUR BRAIN

Introduction

Knowing how to decode nutritional labels is crucial, but what comes next is even more exciting: exploring the buffet of foods that can actively contribute to your cognitive well-being. This chapter will serve as a navigational guide through the culinary landscape, highlighting foods that are not just palatable but also remarkably beneficial for your brain.

The Magical World of Fruits

It's no fairy tale; fruits like blueberries, oranges, and strawberries are packed with antioxidants, Vitamin C, and fiber that benefit your brain. Berries, in particular, are rich in flavonoids, which have been shown to improve memory and delay cognitive aging. Incorporating fruits in your diet can be as simple as tossing them into a morning smoothie or enjoying them as an afternoon snack.

The Nutty Professor: Nuts and Seeds

Einstein may or may not have snacked on walnuts, but you certainly should. Nuts and seeds such as almonds, walnuts, and chia seeds contain essential fatty acids and Vitamin E, which have been linked to less cognitive decline as you age. Some studies suggest that nuts may also enhance brainwave frequencies associated with cognition, healing, and learning. So, go nuts, but in moderation, as they are also calorie-dense.

A Vegetable Affair

If you've been shunning the vegetable section of your grocery store, it's time to rekindle the romance. Leafy greens like kale, spinach, and collards are high in antioxidants, Vitamin K, and folate. These components work together to reduce inflammation and oxidative stress, both of which contribute to cognitive decline. Adding a side of greens to your meals can enrich not only the flavors but also your mental sharpness.

Fishing for Cognition: Seafood and Omega-3s

Seafood, particularly fatty fish like salmon, mackerel, and sardines, are rich in omega-3 fatty acids—known superstars in the realm of cognitive longevity. These fatty acids are essential for brain health, enhancing the structural integrity of brain cells, thereby improving memory and cognitive functions. If you're vegetarian or vegan, fear not; omega-3s are also found in plant sources like flaxseeds and algae oils.

The Egghead Advantage

Eggs have been a subject of culinary debate for years, particularly concerning their cholesterol content. However, they are also a rich source of several nutrients like choline, which is used to produce acetylcholine, a neurotransmitter vital for regulating mood and memory. Incorporating eggs into your diet, therefore, can offer a variety of cognitive benefits. It might just make you an "egghead" in the most flattering sense of the word.

Conclusion

From the orchard of fruits to the fish-filled waters and onto the egg farms, our culinary world offers a smorgasbord of brain-boosting foods. Incorporating these foods into your daily regimen doesn't have to be a tedious affair; rather, it can be a gastronomic adventure with cognitive rewards. The next time you find yourself in a grocery aisle, bewildered by choices, remember that your cart isn't just filled with food; it's stocked with cognitive potential. On to the next chapter, where we explore how the exotic world of spices can also be a treasure trove for your brain.

CHAPTER 6: THE BRAIN'S FAVORITE SPICE: HOW CURCUMIN CAN HELP

Introduction

By now, you're well aware that a host of foods can fuel your brain and keep you sharp. But what if a single spice could offer a myriad of cognitive benefits? In this chapter, we delve into the fascinating world of curcumin, a compound found in turmeric, and its promising role in cognitive longevity.

The Basics of Curcumin: What Is It?

Curcumin is a bright yellow chemical produced by Curcuma longa plants, most commonly known as turmeric. Often used in Asian cooking and traditional medicine, curcumin has gained recent attention in the fields of nutrition and neuroscience for its antioxidant and anti-inflammatory properties. This versatile compound not only brightens your curry but also has the potential to brighten your mind.

Neuroprotective Qualities of Curcumin

Recent research has demonstrated that curcumin might have neuroprotective capabilities. This means it has the potential to guard your brain cells against damage and oxidative stress. Such protective mechanisms could be beneficial in delaying age-related cognitive decline or even neurodegenerative diseases like Alzheimer's. Animal studies have shown that curcumin can enhance the process of clearing amyloid plaques, which are a characteristic feature of Alzheimer's disease.

Anti-Inflammatory and Antioxidant Effects

Chronic inflammation and oxidative stress are known enemies of cognitive function. They accelerate cellular aging and can dampen your mental faculties. Curcumin acts as an anti-inflammatory agent by inhibiting the NF-κB pathway, which plays a pivotal role in inflammatory responses. Its antioxidant properties also neutralize free radicals, thereby reducing oxidative stress. These combined effects make curcumin a candidate for maintaining a healthy, youthful brain.

Mood and Memory: An Uplifting Spice

Though much of the focus is on delaying cognitive decline, let's not overlook the immediate benefits. Some studies suggest that curcumin can be beneficial for mood regulation. It has shown promise in animal models and limited human studies as a natural antidepressant. In particular, curcumin might enhance serotonin and dopamine levels, two neurotransmitters that are heavily involved in mood. On the memory front, curcumin supplementation has demonstrated improvements in working memory and attention in healthy adults, although more research is needed to corroborate these findings.

Incorporating Curcumin Into Your Diet

Given its somewhat pungent and bitter flavor, curcumin is often best enjoyed as a component of broader recipes, such as curries, soups, or even smoothies. It's also available in supplement form but consult with a healthcare provider before starting any new supplement regimen, especially if you're already taking other medications. Note that curcumin is not easily absorbed by the body. Consuming it with black pepper, which contains piperine, can significantly improve its bioavailability.

Conclusion

Curcumin is more than just a spice to add flavor to your meals; it's a potential powerhouse for your brain. From its neuroprotective qualities to its antioxidant and anti-inflammatory effects, this remarkable compound shows promise in maintaining cognitive health and even uplifting your mood. Though research is ongoing, the preliminary results make a compelling case for including curcumin in your cognitive longevity toolkit. Consider incorporating this golden spice into your diet to potentially add some luster to your golden years.

CHAPTER 7: SIP TO SHARPEN: THE BENEFITS OF HYDRATION

When it comes to cognitive longevity, the importance of hydration is a topic that often takes a backseat to more glamorous subjects like antioxidants, vitamins, or brain-boosting superfoods. Yet, the elixir of life—water—holds transformative power for your cognitive capabilities. In this chapter, we'll delve into the science of hydration and cognition, explore the best liquids for your brain, and offer tips on staying well-hydrated.

The Cognitive Chemistry of Water

Your brain is approximately 75% water. Dehydration, even mild, affects the brain's structure and functions. When your brain cells lack adequate water, they work less efficiently, leading to cognitive deficits like impaired attention, memory, and executive functions. Neurotransmission, which facilitates the communication between your neurons, is also heavily dependent on proper hydration. Therefore, water is not just a physiological need but a cognitive enhancer, lubricating the gears of your mental machinery.

Hydration Metrics: How Much is Enough?

The general recommendation to drink eight 8-ounce glasses of water per day is a decent starting point, but it's far from one-size-fits-all. Factors like age, activity level, and climate all contribute to your specific hydration needs. Focusing on the color of your urine can provide a more tailored guideline; a pale yellow signifies well-hydrated status. But don't just sip when you're thirsty. Thirst is a lagging indicator of hydration status; by the time you feel thirsty, you may already be mildly dehydrated.

Water Alternatives: Friend or Foe?

Not all liquids are created equal when it comes to hydration. While water is the gold standard, other beverages can also contribute to your hydration levels. Herbal teas and coconut water are good alternatives. On the other hand, caffeinated drinks and alcohol can lead to dehydration. Be cautious of sugary drinks as well; they might hydrate you initially, but the sugar content can lead to other cognitive issues. Stick with water and other low-sugar options to ensure your cognitive wheel keeps turning smoothly.

The Electrolyte Equation

Electrolytes like sodium, potassium, and magnesium play a crucial role in maintaining fluid balance within cells. When discussing hydration, it's not just the water but also these vital elements that matter. Foods rich in natural electrolytes—such as bananas, avocados, and spinach—can boost your hydration status. Some people opt for electrolyte-infused water, especially after intense physical activity, but for most, a balanced diet should suffice for keeping electrolyte levels in check.

Practical Hydration Hacks for Cognitive Longevity

Staying well-hydrated doesn't have to be a chore. Here are some actionable tips:

- Keep a refillable water bottle with you at all times.
- Infuse water with natural flavors like lemon, cucumber, or mint to add variety.
- Use reminders or apps to track your hydration levels.
- Incorporate water-rich foods like watermelon, cucumber, and oranges into your diet.
- Balance your beverage choices, leaning more towards herbal teas and pure water, and limiting caffeinated or sugary drinks.

In summary, the road to cognitive longevity is not just paved with nutrient-dense foods; it also runs along rivers of well-balanced hydration. Recognizing the profound influence of hydration on cognitive functions, and taking proactive steps to stay hydrated, can significantly aid in maintaining your mental acuity as you age. So the next time you're feeling mentally sluggish, consider reaching for a glass of water—it might just be the cognitive pick-me-up you need.

CHAPTER 8: THE SUGAR CONUNDRUM: SWEET BUT NOT SO INNOCENT

Introduction

Ah, sugar—the siren song in most culinary operas, the sweet symphony that dances across our taste buds. As alluring as it may be, the repercussions of indulging in sugar can reverberate far beyond those extra inches on your waistline. It turns out, sugar can sabotage your cognitive function in more ways than one. So, let's peel back the sugar-coated curtain and examine what's really going on in that sweet-loving brain of yours.

The Biochemical Backstage: Sugar and the Brain

Contrary to popular belief, not all sugars are demonic entities waiting to pounce on your cognitive well-being. Glucose, for example, is the brain's primary source of energy. However, the issue arises when excessive refined sugars enter the equation. Refined sugars, like sucrose and high fructose corn syrup, have a knack for causing a rapid spike and subsequent drop in blood glucose levels. This sugar rollercoaster wreaks havoc on neurotransmitter regulation, which is critical for mood, focus, and memory. Moreover, these dramatic swings can cause mental fog and leave you with that infamous "sugar crash," impacting your cognitive resilience in the process.

The Inflammation Equation

Inflammation is your body's innate response to injury or illness, but when it comes to sugar, the situation can escalate into chronic inflammation, a potential threat to cognitive longevity. Studies indicate that high sugar consumption can trigger a domino effect, culminating in an inflamed brain. This is no small matter as chronic neuroinflammation is linked to a variety of cognitive disorders, including Alzheimer's disease and other forms of dementia.

Sugar's Assault on the Microbiome

By now, you're aware that the gut-brain axis is a two-way informational highway, affecting everything from your mood to your memory. But what role does sugar play? Unfortunately, refined sugars are notorious for fueling the growth of harmful gut bacteria, thereby skewing the balance of your microbiome. These bacterial imbalances can result in the production of neurotoxic metabolites and increase the permeability of the gut lining, known colloquially as "leaky gut." Consequently, this compromises the blood-brain barrier and allows harmful substances to enter the brain, often leading to cognitive decline.

The Cognitive Tax of Insulin Resistance

Frequent high sugar consumption can also lead to insulin resistance, a condition where cells in your body don't respond well to insulin. This is a particularly grave concern for your brain. Insulin plays an integral role in synaptic plasticity, learning, and memory formation. When your brain's insulin receptors are compromised, it may lead to impaired cognitive function and even elevate your risk for neurodegenerative diseases.

Curbing the Sugar Seduction

Unraveling from the sweet grasp of sugar is no easy feat, but it's crucial for safeguarding your cognitive longevity. Start by identifying hidden sources of sugar in processed foods; you'd be surprised how much sugar is lurking in everyday items like bread, pasta sauces, and even so-called "healthy" snacks. Next, venture into natural sweeteners like stevia or monk fruit, which have less of an impact on blood sugar levels. Remember, moderation is key; a little sweetness is okay as long as it's not overpowering your plate or your brain.

Conclusion

The love affair between sugar and modern diets is a complicated entanglement, fraught with highs and lows, not just for your body but also for your brain. By understanding how refined sugars can adversely affect your cognitive performance and long-term brain health, you can make informed choices. It's not about deprivation but about elevating your nutritional game to preserve that sharp, agile mind of yours. And when you can make that compromise, the benefits aren't just sweet; they're enduringly profound.

CHAPTER 9: THE PROTEIN PERSPECTIVE: BUILDING BLOCKS OF THE BRAIN

Introduction

By now, you're well-versed in the evils of sugar and the virtues of hydration and spices like curcumin when it comes to brain health. But have you ever wondered about the significance of protein in this cognitive symphony? Prepare to uncover the role of protein as an essential pillar for building and maintaining a sharper, resilient mind.

Proteins: More Than Muscle Food

Commonly associated with bodybuilders and athletes, proteins serve a broader biological purpose. Each protein molecule is a complex structure made up of amino acids, which are the real heroes behind neurotransmission and other brain functions. Neurotransmitters like dopamine and serotonin, responsible for mood and emotional regulation, are built from amino acids. In simple terms, insufficient protein intake could dampen your spirits and affect your focus.

Essential Amino Acids and Brain Function

Not all amino acids are created equal. While your body can manufacture some, called non-essential amino acids, there are nine "essential" ones you must obtain from your diet. These are crucial for producing neurochemicals that govern aspects of cognition, from memory to executive functions like decision-making. Foods rich in essential amino acids include lean meats, fish, dairy, and legumes. Neglect these, and you may experience subpar cognitive performance.

Quality Over Quantity: Bioavailability

When discussing protein for cognitive longevity, it's not just about piling up steak on your plate. The concept of "bioavailability" refers to how efficiently your body can use the protein you consume. Animal sources like eggs, chicken, and fish generally have high bioavailability, meaning your body can readily absorb and use their amino acids. Plant-based proteins like lentils, chickpeas, and tofu are also good but often require pairing with other proteins to form a complete amino acid profile.

The Danger of Overdoing It

While protein is pivotal, an overload is counterproductive. Excessive protein intake can strain the kidneys and even offset the brain's delicate neurochemical balance. Elevated levels of certain amino acids could compete with others like tryptophan, which is essential for serotonin production. This imbalance may potentially lead to mood swings and cognitive inconsistencies.

Protein Timing: Spreading It Out

As with most nutrients, timing your protein intake can also influence cognitive performance. Consuming protein in excessive amounts at one go won't guarantee better brain function.

Spreading your protein intake throughout the day ensures a steady supply of essential amino acids, aiding in consistent neurotransmission and cognitive function. Include some form of protein in each meal and consider protein-rich snacks like Greek yogurt or a handful of almonds between meals.

Conclusion

In the orchestra of nutrients that contribute to cognitive longevity, protein plays a starring role. It's not merely the building block of muscles but of neurochemicals that make mental acuity possible. Striking the right balance of quality protein, sourced from a mix of animal and plant foods, is key to maintaining a consistent cognitive performance. As you journey through your dietary changes, let protein be the steadfast friend who enriches your cognitive wellbeing without overwhelming it.

CHAPTER 10: VITAMIN VELOCITY: SPEEDING UP MENTAL ACUITY

Introduction

Vitamins are often hailed as little marvels of nature that contribute to various bodily functions, from boosting immunity to promoting healthy skin. When it comes to brain health and cognitive longevity, the role of vitamins becomes even more intriguing. Let's unpack the enigma surrounding the importance of vitamins for mental acuity and how they can act as accelerants in the quest for cognitive longevity.

The Role of B Vitamins in Brain Health

Among the vitamins, the B group stands out for its direct and potent influence on brain function. Vitamin B12, for instance, plays a critical role in the production of red blood cells, which in turn enhances oxygen delivery to the brain. A lack of B12 can result in cognitive impairments and even mood disorders like depression. Other B vitamins like B6 and folic acid also contribute to neurotransmitter synthesis, the key chemical messengers that ensure smooth brain function.

Vitamin D: The Sunshine Vitamin

Vitamin D has become something of a celebrity in the vitamin world, thanks to its range of health benefits. While you may associate it with strong bones, it also has notable impacts on the brain. Studies have shown that Vitamin D receptors are present throughout the brain, and deficiencies in this vitamin are linked with conditions like Alzheimer's disease and cognitive decline. Moreover, vitamin D aids in the regulation of various neurotransmitters like dopamine and serotonin, which affect mood and cognition.

Vitamin C: More Than Just an Immunity Booster

Vitamin C is often pigeonholed as an immunity warrior, but it does more than just fend off the common cold. This vitamin is a potent antioxidant that protects brain cells from oxidative damage, thereby playing a role in the prevention of neurodegenerative diseases. It also promotes the synthesis of collagen, a protein that makes up the protective sheath around neurons, enhancing neural integrity.

Vitamin E: The Guardian of Membranes

Fat-soluble vitamin E is renowned for its antioxidant properties, particularly in protecting the integrity of cell membranes. Since brain cells have a high fat content, they are susceptible to oxidative stress, a condition vitamin E can counteract effectively. Studies indicate that higher levels of vitamin E intake may be correlated with better cognitive performance and a lower risk of diseases like Alzheimer's.

Vitamin K: The Unsung Hero

Vitamin K is often overlooked, but it plays a vital role in brain health by aiding in the regulation of calcium within the bones and the bloodstream. Imbalanced calcium levels can lead to neural deterioration, emphasizing the importance of vitamin K in preserving cognitive function. It also plays a role in the synthesis of sphingolipids, a type of lipid that is abundantly present in brain cell membranes.

Conclusion

Vitamins are more than just supplementary nutrients; they are vital players in the grand arena of cognitive function. From the B vitamins that aid neurotransmitter synthesis to the fat-soluble vitamins that protect neural membranes, these micronutrients are integral to maintaining mental acuity as you age. Incorporating a diet rich in these vitamins can indeed act as a catalyst in your journey towards cognitive longevity. Consider them your small, yet powerful, allies in achieving a sharper, more resilient mind.

CHAPTER 11: MINDING YOUR GUT: THE BRAIN-GUT CONNECTION

Introduction

Ah, the gut—a place commonly associated with digestion, intuition, and the occasional belly laugh. But would you believe that this unassuming part of your body holds significant sway over your brain? Let's unravel the intricate connection between your gut and cognitive function.

The Microbiome Marvel

Your gut isn't just a food processing unit; it's also home to trillions of microorganisms known as the microbiome. This microscopic community includes bacteria, viruses, and fungi, which aid in digestion, immunity, and shockingly, even cognitive function. Emerging research shows a two-way street of communication between the gut and the brain, humorously dubbed the "gut-brain axis."

Neurotransmitters: The Chemical Messengers

You've probably heard of neurotransmitters like serotonin and dopamine, usually in the context of mood and mental well-being. Here's a gut punch of a fact: a majority of serotonin, often called the "feel-good" hormone, is produced in the gut. These neurotransmitters don't just stick around in your belly, waiting for a bus to nowhere; they communicate with the brain, influencing your emotions, memory, and decision-making abilities.

Inflammation and Cognitive Decline

Inflammation is your body's natural response to injury or infection, but chronic inflammation is a party crasher nobody likes. It has been linked to cognitive decline and a host of neurodegenerative diseases. Your gut plays a leading role in controlling inflammation. An imbalance in gut bacteria can tip the scale, resulting in inflammation that goes beyond local and enters systemic circulation, affecting brain health.

Food Choices for a Balanced Gut-Brain Axis

Choosing foods rich in probiotics like yogurt, kefir, and fermented foods such as sauerkraut and kimchi can bring balance to your gut flora. Prebiotics—non-digestible food components—also deserve some love. They serve as food for the good bacteria in your gut. Sources include garlic, onions, and whole grains. Let's not forget fiber; it isn't just for regularity. A high-fiber diet supports a healthy microbiome, which, in turn, can contribute to improved mental clarity.

Beyond Nutrition: Lifestyle Choices and Stress Management

Stress not only frazzles your nerves but also unsettles your gut. Stress management techniques such as mindfulness meditation, adequate sleep, and regular exercise can go a long way in maintaining a harmonious gut-brain relationship. It's not just what you eat, but how you live that contributes to cognitive longevity.

Conclusion

Forget "you are what you eat" for a moment and consider this: you think how you eat. The gut may be miles away from the brain, but they're in constant chatter, and that conversation has profound implications for cognitive longevity. Nourishing your gut with smart food choices and a balanced lifestyle could very well be a ticket to a sharper, more resilient mind as you age.

CHAPTER 12: PORTION CONTROL: HOW MUCH IS JUST RIGHT?

Introduction

When it comes to cognitive longevity, the kind of food you eat isn't the only game in town; the size of your portions also plays a critical role. This chapter will help you navigate the labyrinth of portion sizes, offering strategies to find that "Goldilocks Zone" where the amount is "just right" for your brain's needs.

Decoding the Portion Puzzle

Determining the right portion size can be a complicated affair. Labels and diet plans may give the illusion of straightforward guidance, but they often overlook individual variances like metabolism, activity level, and even cognitive demand. However, modern nutrition science offers some universally applicable rules.

For proteins, a serving size roughly equal to the palm of your hand is generally recommended. In terms of vegetables, more is almost always better—aim for at least two fist-sized servings per meal. As for fats and carbs, a thumb-sized portion of fats and a cupped-hand portion of carbs usually hit the mark. These are simple approximations but serve as a useful starting point.

The Science of Satiety

Feeling full isn't just about filling your stomach; it's a complex process involving a symphony of hormones and neurological signals. Foods high in protein, fiber, and healthy fats tend to be more satiating. Moreover, they often have a lower glycemic index, meaning they release sugar into the bloodstream slowly, providing sustained energy and focus. This is particularly useful in maintaining cognitive functions throughout the day.

Understanding the science of satiety can also help in making better portion choices. Consuming a small protein-rich snack between meals, for example, can help keep your cognitive gears lubricated without the risk of overeating during mealtime.

Mindful Eating: The Conscious Approach to Portions

If you eat while distracted, you're less likely to pay attention to portion sizes. Mindful eating—focusing on each bite and savoring the textures and flavors—can help you become aware of your satiety cues. This helps in stopping when you're full rather than when your plate is empty. It turns out that the brain takes about 20 minutes to register fullness, so eating slowly can be a wise strategy to avoid overconsumption and the subsequent cognitive sluggishness.

Portion Distortion: Societal Influences and Their Pitfalls

If you've ever dined out, you'll know that restaurant portions can be ludicrously large. Unfortunately, these super-sized servings have skewed our perception of what is "normal." This phenomenon, known as "portion distortion," has serious implications for cognitive health. Studies show that excessive caloric intake, even if only occasional, can induce oxidative stress and inflammation, both of which are detrimental to cognitive function.

Plan Ahead: Strategies for Perfect Portions

Meal prepping can be a lifesaver when it comes to maintaining portion control. By setting aside time to plan and prepare your meals for the week, you eliminate the guesswork. You also limit the opportunities for impulsive, less cognitive-friendly choices. Useful tools include kitchen scales, measuring cups, and pre-portioned containers to ensure consistency.

When dining out, consider sharing dishes or immediately boxing up half of your meal to avoid the trap of cleaning your plate. These proactive strategies can safeguard against the cognitive pitfalls of overconsumption.

Conclusion

While the types of food you eat significantly influence cognitive longevity, how much you eat is equally vital. By decoding the portion puzzle, understanding the science of satiety, practicing mindful eating, and planning ahead, you set the stage for a nourished and agile mind as you age. After all, the most elegant solutions are often about striking the right balance.

CHAPTER 13: CARB-LOADED OR CARB-LIMITED?

Introduction

Carbohydrates, often shorthand for both comfort food and calories, get mixed reviews when it comes to their impact on cognition. Are they brain fuel, or do they simply fuel debates about their true nature? Let's delve into the complex relationship between carbs and cognitive health.

The Basic Biochemistry of Carbohydrates

Carbohydrates are classified into three categories: simple carbohydrates (sugars), complex carbohydrates (starches), and fiber. Your body converts all digestible carbohydrates into glucose, which is essential for brain function. In fact, the brain is the primary consumer of glucose in your body. That said, not all carbohydrates are created equal. While the brain relies heavily on glucose, the type and quality of carbs you consume can have contrasting effects on cognitive function.

The Glycemic Index: A Cognitive Compass

The Glycemic Index (GI) measures how quickly a food causes blood sugar to rise. Foods with a high GI, like white bread and sugary drinks, cause rapid spikes in blood sugar and have been linked to cognitive decline over time. On the other hand, low-GI foods such as whole grains, fruits, and vegetables, lead to a slower release of glucose, offering a steadier source of energy for the brain. Adopting a low-GI diet has been linked with improvements in memory, attention, and overall mental performance.

Carbs and Mood: An Emotional Affair

You might have noticed that when you eat carbs, particularly the comforting simple ones like cookies or pasta, you momentarily feel happier. This short-lived bliss is due to serotonin, a neurotransmitter that elevates mood. However, such mood lifts are often followed by a crash, leading to an emotional rollercoaster that's not conducive to cognitive stability. Thus, opting for carbs that are rich in fiber and have a lower GI can help stabilize mood, indirectly aiding cognitive function.

Carb-Limited Diets: Ketones and Cognition

Ketogenic diets, which are low in carbs and high in fats, shift the body's energy source from glucose to ketones. Initial studies suggest that this metabolic state, called ketosis, may have neuroprotective effects and could even improve cognitive function in individuals with neurodegenerative disorders like Alzheimer's. However, the long-term implications of a ketogenic diet on cognitive health are still under exploration. Plus, being in a constant state of ketosis may not be suitable for everyone and can have other health implications.

Fine-Tuning Your Carb Intake

Determining the right amount and type of carbs for cognitive longevity involves more than counting calories or going low-carb for the sake of it. The key is balance. A diet rich in complex carbohydrates from whole grains, fruits, and vegetables, balanced with protein and healthy fats, could offer the brain a sustained supply of energy. It's about making intelligent carb choices rather than boycotting carbs altogether.

Conclusion

The debate on carbs and cognition is not about vilifying or championing carbs, but understanding their nuanced role in brain health. From the Glycemic Index to ketogenic diets, it's evident that not all carbs have the same impact on your cognitive well-being. In a world where extreme dieting is often in vogue, remember that it's the thoughtful selection and balanced intake of carbs that might just keep your mind sharp as a tack as you age.

CHAPTER 14: FISHY BUSINESS: THE ROLE OF OMEGA-3S

Introduction

For some, the notion of "fishy business" might conjure images of suspect deals or less-than-transparent operations. In this context, however, we're talking about the kind of fishy business that's decidedly above board and beneficial for your brain: Omega-3 fatty acids. Get ready to dive deep into the sea of scientific evidence to discover why Omega-3s are known as the "brain food."

Unveiling Omega-3s: The Basics

Omega-3 fatty acids are a class of essential fatty acids, which means the body can't produce them on its own and must acquire them through diet. These fatty acids play critical roles in various physiological functions, including cell membrane structure and anti-inflammatory processes. The main types of Omega-3s are ALA (alpha-linolenic acid), EPA (eicosapentaenoic acid), and DHA (docosahexaenoic acid).

Neurological Nourishment: Omega-3s and Brain Health

The brain comprises nearly 60% fat, and a large portion of it is omega-3 fatty acids, particularly DHA. DHA contributes to the fluidity of cell membranes, which is crucial for synaptic transmission—the way your brain cells (neurons) communicate. This cell communication is foundational for cognitive functions like learning, memory, and reasoning. Research has also found a significant correlation between adequate levels of Omega-3s and decreased risks of age-related cognitive decline, Alzheimer's, and depression.

From Sea to Brain: Best Food Sources

When it comes to sourcing Omega-3s, fatty fish reign supreme. Salmon, mackerel, and sardines are among the most Omega-3-rich foods. If you're vegetarian or vegan, fear not; you can also obtain Omega-3s from algae oil, walnuts, flaxseeds, and chia seeds, although these primarily contain ALA, which the body then needs to convert to DHA and EPA. However, it's worth noting that the conversion rate is inefficient, meaning you may need to consume higher amounts.

Serving Size and Supplements: Getting the Right Amount

The recommended daily intake of Omega-3s varies by age and individual health considerations, but a general guideline is about 250–500 mg combined EPA and DHA. It can be a challenge to meet this quota through diet alone, especially if you're not a fan of fish. In such cases, Omega-3 supplements might be your ally. When opting for supplements, look for those that are third-party tested for purity to avoid possible contaminants like heavy metals.

The Omega-3 Debate: Controversies and Considerations

While Omega-3s have been touted for their health benefits, they are not a magical cure for all cognitive ailments. Some research has produced inconsistent results on their effectiveness in improving memory and cognitive performance. Moreover, Omega-3 supplements may interact with certain medications or exacerbate conditions like prostate cancer. Therefore, it's crucial to consult healthcare professionals for personalized advice.

Conclusion

Navigating the world of nutritional neuroscience may sometimes feel like you're lost at sea, but understanding the value of Omega-3s can be your compass to more vibrant cognitive health. These essential fatty acids, abundant in certain fish and other food sources, are cornerstones of cellular function and anti-inflammatory processes, directly impacting your brain's performance and long-term wellness. While they're not a panacea, they're a critical part of your dietary strategy for cognitive longevity. So go ahead, engage in this kind of fishy business; your brain will thank you.

CHAPTER 15: TIMING IS EVERYTHING: WHEN TO EAT FOR COGNITIVE POWER

Introduction

Your brain's cognitive functions are not just influenced by what you eat, but also when you eat it. This chapter dives into the intriguing world of meal timing, exploring how it can be optimized to sustain mental acuity and fend off age-related cognitive decline.

The Circadian Rhythm and Cognitive Performance

Most biological functions, including those in your brain, are regulated by a 24-hour internal clock known as the circadian rhythm. During certain periods, your brain is more alert and capable of handling tasks that require memory, attention, and problem-solving. It turns out that this rhythm is also influenced by your eating patterns. Consuming food at consistent times can help synchronize your body's clock, which in turn can positively affect cognitive functions.

Breakfast: To Skip or Not to Skip

The debate around breakfast and its importance has been lengthy.

For cognitive performance, however, several studies suggest that a balanced morning meal can improve memory and attention spans throughout the day. Skipping breakfast, on the other hand, may lead to decreased cognitive performance, particularly in complex tasks. Therefore, a nutrient-rich breakfast that includes elements like whole grains, lean protein, and fruit could be the key to kick-starting your brain in the morning.

Late-Night Snacking: A Cognitive Faux Pas?

Eating late at night isn't just problematic for your waistline; it could also affect your brain's functionality. The digestive process requires energy, and when you eat right before sleeping, your body has to juggle between digestion and restorative processes that are vital for cognitive health. This juggling act can result in reduced quality of sleep and impaired memory. Additionally, late-night eating can disrupt your circadian rhythm, potentially throwing off your mental sharpness the next day.

Intermittent Fasting and Cognitive Benefits

Intermittent fasting, the practice of alternating between periods of eating and fasting, has been shown to have various health benefits, including potential cognitive improvements. The primary mechanism behind this is thought to be autophagy, a cellular "cleanup" process that gets activated during fasting. This process removes damaged cells and regenerates new ones, contributing to improved mental acuity. However, the extent to which intermittent fasting benefits cognitive function is still under research, and it may not be suitable for everyone.

Timing Nutrients for Cognitive Peaks

Certain nutrients are known for their cognitive-enhancing properties, such as Omega-3 fatty acids, antioxidants, and specific amino acids like tyrosine. The timing of consuming these nutrients can be crucial. For instance, amino acids like tyrosine are precursors to neurotransmitters that influence mood and focus. Eating a meal rich in these amino acids a couple of hours before a cognitively demanding task may offer a performance boost. Similarly, antioxidants like those found in berries could be consumed throughout the day for sustained cognitive support.

Conclusion

As it turns out, timing really is everything, especially when it comes to your cognitive performance. Synchronizing your meals with your body's internal clock can have a notable impact on mental acuity. Whether it's making sure not to skip breakfast or avoiding late-night munchies, the when of eating is a factor that shouldn't be overlooked in your quest for cognitive longevity. So, set your watches and align your meals; your brain will thank you for it.

CHAPTER 16: ANTIOXIDANT ARSENAL: FOODS THAT FIGHT COGNITIVE DECLINE

Antioxidants—often buzzwords in health circles, but rarely understood in depth—are your brain's natural bodyguards. They fight against oxidative stress, a villain in the narrative of aging and cognitive decline. This chapter delves into the role of antioxidants in cognitive longevity and presents you with a list of foods rich in these natural defenders.

What Are Antioxidants and Why Does the Brain Need Them?

Oxidative stress occurs when there's an imbalance between free radicals and antioxidants in the body. Free radicals are unstable atoms that can damage cells, contributing to aging and diseases. The brain is particularly susceptible to oxidative stress due to its high consumption of oxygen and its abundant fatty acids which are prone to oxidation. Antioxidants come to the rescue by neutralizing these free radicals, thereby preventing cellular damage. In the context of cognitive longevity, antioxidants may slow down age-related brain diseases like Alzheimer's and preserve neural integrity.

The Fruitful Offense: Berries and Citrus

Berries such as blueberries, raspberries, and strawberries are the jewels of the antioxidant kingdom. A study published in the "Journal of Agricultural and Food Chemistry" pointed out that berries might help to improve memory and cognitive performance. Berries are rich in antioxidants like flavonoids, anthocyanins, and vitamin C, making them an excellent choice for brain health. Similarly, citrus fruits like oranges, grapefruits, and lemons are high in vitamin C, another powerful antioxidant.

The Veggie Defense: Spinach, Kale, and Broccoli

Green leafy vegetables, especially spinach, kale, and broccoli, are filled with antioxidants such as lutein, zeaxanthin, and vitamin E. Lutein and zeaxanthin accumulate in the brain and could possibly provide cognitive benefits. Vitamin E is particularly noteworthy because of its ability to cross the blood-brain barrier, making it especially effective in combating oxidative stress in the brain.

Nutty Guardians: Almonds and Walnuts

Nuts are nature's bite-sized brain boosters. Almonds are a rich source of vitamin E, while walnuts contain a variety of antioxidants, including ellagic acid, which has been shown to protect against oxidative stress. Additionally, walnuts are one of the few plant sources of Omega-3 fatty acids, which, as discussed in a previous chapter, are crucial for brain health.

Liquid Lifelines: Green Tea and Red Wine

Polyphenols found in green tea have antioxidative and neuroprotective properties. One of the most well-researched polyphenols in green tea is epigallocatechin gallate (EGCG), which has been found to protect neuronal cells. Red wine, when consumed in moderation, contains resveratrol, a type of antioxidant that has shown promise in promoting longevity and cognitive health. However, the key is moderation; excessive alcohol consumption can negate these benefits and introduce a host of other health problems.

Spice it Up: Turmeric and Cinnamon

Turmeric contains curcumin, a potent antioxidant and anti-inflammatory agent. Curcumin is of particular interest in the field of cognitive neuroscience due to its potential to reduce symptoms of Alzheimer's disease. Cinnamon, on the other hand, contains antioxidants like polyphenols and has anti-inflammatory properties. The inclusion of these spices in your meals can be a flavorful and effective way to boost your antioxidant intake.

In summary, antioxidants are invaluable allies in your quest for cognitive longevity. Incorporating a variety of antioxidant-rich foods into your diet can make a world of difference in your brain health. From juicy berries to green tea, your choices are as delicious as they are beneficial. Make your kitchen a bastion of cognitive resilience by stocking it with these antioxidant powerhouses.

CHAPTER 17: MINDFUL MUNCHING: THE PRACTICE OF MINDFUL EATING

Introduction

We often eat to satiate hunger or please our taste buds, but how often do we really engage with our meals? Mindfulness—being fully present in the moment—extends far beyond the yoga mat or meditation cushion, right into our dining tables. In this chapter, we explore how mindful eating can influence not just our digestion, but also our cognitive well-being.

The Science Behind Mindful Eating and Cognition

Mindful eating originates from the broader concept of mindfulness—a mental state achieved by concentrating on the current moment. By bringing mindfulness to eating, we engage our senses, making the eating experience richer and more enjoyable. Scientific studies indicate that mindful eating can have an impact on cognitive functions like focus, memory, and emotional control.

For example, a 2014 study published in the journal Psychological Reports indicated that mindfulness could positively affect cognitive flexibility—a mental characteristic associated with problem-solving and adapting to new situations. If you're eating mindfully, you're practicing cognitive flexibility by adapting to each unique meal experience.

How to Eat Mindfully

Let's break down how to actually practice mindful eating:

- Turn Off Distractions: Begin by eliminating distractions like the TV, smartphone, or even reading material.
- Sit Down: Eating while standing or walking can hamper your ability to focus on the food.
- Smell the Aroma: Take a moment to appreciate the smell of the food, which sets the stage for the digestive process.
- Chew Slowly: Each bite should be chewed multiple times, which assists in both digestion and allows you to savor each flavor.
- Taste Thoroughly: Take note of each flavor—sweet, sour, bitter, salty, umami—and how they change as you chew.

Remember, it's not just what you eat but also how you eat that impacts your cognition.

Mindful Eating and Portion Control

Being aware of each bite helps you recognize when you are actually full, thereby aiding in portion control. When you eat quickly, your body doesn't have the time to send fullness signals to your brain, often leading to overeating. Overeating, especially when it involves unhealthy foods rich in saturated fats and sugar, can negatively impact cognitive function. Through mindful eating, you can be more in tune with your body's signals, allowing for better portion control that aligns with your cognitive longevity goals.

Mindful Eating for Improved Mental Health

Interestingly, the benefits of mindful eating also extend to mental health. Anxiety and depression are closely related to cognitive decline. Mindful eating forces you to focus on the present, serving as a form of meditation that reduces stress. A 2016 study published in the journal Mindfulness and Eating Behavior demonstrated that individuals who practiced mindful eating reported less incidence of depressive symptoms and exhibited better cognitive function compared to those who didn't.

Emotional Eating and Mindfulness

We often reach for comfort foods when we're stressed, sad, or even bored. This type of emotional eating can be detrimental to both our waistline and brain health. The practice of mindful eating encourages you to pause and question the reason behind your hunger. Are you eating because you're genuinely hungry, or is it an emotional response? By taking this moment to assess your emotional state, you can make better dietary choices that are in line with your cognitive longevity goals.

Conclusion

Mindful eating is not just a fashionable term; it is a practical and scientifically supported strategy to enhance cognitive function. It allows for better portion control, improved mental health, and offers a tool to combat emotional eating. So the next time you sit down for a meal, remember to engage your senses fully, savor each bite, and be aware of your body's signals. By doing so, you're not just nourishing your body; you're also feeding your mind.

CHAPTER 18: MOVE TO THINK: EXERCISE AS COGNITIVE FUEL

Introduction

It's clear that the foods you eat can power your brain, but did you ever consider that pumping your muscles might actually juice up your neurons? This chapter delves into the lesser-acknowledged sibling of diet in the cognitive longevity equation: exercise.

The Science of Exercise and Brain Function

Once dismissed as mere "brain sweat," exercise is now hailed as an invaluable component for cognitive health. It enhances neural connectivity, improves mental clarity, and even fosters the growth of new neurons—a process known as neurogenesis. Unlike your muscles, which have a limited ability to regenerate, your brain can actually produce new cells when you exercise. Think of it as a cerebral renovation with every lap, squat, or yoga pose.

The Cardio-Cognitive Connection

If you're looking to get the maximum cognitive bang for your exercise buck, cardiovascular workouts should be your go-to. Aerobic exercises like running, cycling, and swimming are stellar at elevating your heart rate and, subsequently, your blood flow.

This means more oxygen and nutrients for your brain, leading to better performance in tasks that require memory, attention, and problem-solving skills. One particularly intriguing study found that aerobic exercise could even increase the size of the hippocampus—the brain area associated with memory and spatial navigation. A larger hippocampus is like having a more expansive mental library, offering more space to store memories and navigate complex problems.

Exercise and Neurotransmitters

Exercise isn't just a physical challenge; it's a biochemical ballet in your brain. Physical activity prompts the release of neurotransmitters like dopamine, serotonin, and norepinephrine, which play pivotal roles in mood regulation, focus, and even resilience to stress. Interestingly, these are the same neurotransmitters targeted by many antidepressant medications. But unlike pharmaceuticals, exercise doesn't come with a long list of potential side effects—unless you count a toned physique and better mental acuity as "side effects."

Timing and Types of Exercise

While any exercise is better than none, the timing and type of exercise you choose can have varying effects on your cognitive performance. Morning workouts, for example, can kickstart your mental engines for the day ahead, while evening exercise may help you unwind and prepare for a restorative sleep. As for the type, a blend of aerobic exercise, strength training, and flexibility exercises like yoga or Pilates offers a holistic approach to cognitive health. The variety not only keeps you engaged but also ensures you're targeting different aspects of cognition.

Exercise as a Cognitive Lifestyle

It's easy to pigeonhole exercise as a mere physical endeavor, but reframe it as part of your cognitive lifestyle, and you'll be more motivated to stick with it. After all, you're not just working out to look good; you're training to think better. Making exercise a part of your daily routine doesn't just mean a healthier body; it translates to a sharper, more agile mind, capable of tackling challenges with finesse.

Conclusion

Exercise is a potent, often underestimated tool for enhancing cognitive function. From its ability to stimulate neurotransmitter activity to its role in fostering new neural connections, regular physical activity is every bit as crucial as diet for maintaining a sharp mind as you age. So, the next time you find yourself debating whether to hit the gym or laze on the couch, remember: you're not just shaping your muscles; you're sculpting your mind.

CHAPTER 19: CAFFEINE AND COGNITION: A LOVE-HATE RELATIONSHIP

The aroma of freshly brewed coffee wafts through the air, tantalizing your senses. There's a sense of ritual, comfort, and—let's face it—necessity in a cup of joe that heralds the start of a new day. For many, caffeine is the elixir that not only lifts the morning fog but also sharpens the mental blade. Yet, questions abound: Is caffeine the unsung hero of cognitive longevity, or does it merely masquerade as a friend while quietly undermining your brain's future? In this chapter, we'll explore this intricate dance between caffeine and cognition.

The Perks of Caffeine

You've probably noticed that your first cup of coffee or tea puts you in a state of heightened alertness. That's because caffeine is a natural stimulant. It acts as an adenosine receptor antagonist, meaning it blocks the function of adenosine, a neurotransmitter that promotes sleep and relaxation. By doing so, caffeine indirectly increases the release of other neurotransmitters like dopamine and norepinephrine, leading to improved mood, better concentration, and increased alertness.

Several studies suggest that moderate caffeine consumption can aid cognitive functions. For instance, caffeine has been found to improve performance in tasks that require attention, enhance short-term memory, and even boost physical endurance by acting on the central nervous system. And it's not just a short-term crutch; research indicates that regular, moderate caffeine intake might be associated with a lower risk of Alzheimer's and Parkinson's diseases.

The Downsides: Caffeine's Dark Roast

However, it's not all sips and roses. While caffeine can enhance certain aspects of cognition, it's far from a silver bullet. Excessive caffeine consumption has been linked to increased anxiety, sleep disturbances, and even depressive symptoms. Caffeine can also have a diuretic effect, potentially leading to dehydration, which as we learned in Chapter 7, can be detrimental to cognitive performance.

Another aspect worth noting is caffeine's half-life, which can range from 3 to 5 hours. This means that if you consume a cup of coffee late in the afternoon, a substantial amount of caffeine could still be in your system come bedtime, disrupting sleep quality and the restorative processes that are crucial for cognitive longevity.

Individual Responses and Genetics

Not everyone metabolizes caffeine in the same way. Some people are genetically predisposed to process caffeine quickly, while others are slow metabolizers. For fast metabolizers, caffeine can offer most of its benefits without many of its drawbacks. On the other hand, slow metabolizers may experience increased heart rate, higher levels of anxiety, and a higher susceptibility to the negative sleep-related side-effects. Therefore, understanding your individual tolerance to caffeine can guide you in harnessing its cognitive benefits while minimizing its potential downsides.

Alternatives and Moderation

If you're looking to reduce caffeine intake but still crave a cognitive boost, there are alternatives. Substances like L-theanine, found in green tea, have been shown to improve focus and relaxation, often without the jitters that accompany a caffeine buzz. Additionally, herbs like ginseng and rhodiola have also been touted for their cognitive-enhancing benefits.

When it comes to caffeine, moderation seems to be key. For most people, sticking to around 200-400 mg of caffeine per day (roughly equivalent to 2-4 cups of brewed coffee) seems to offer cognitive benefits without too many drawbacks.

Conclusion

The relationship between caffeine and cognition is complex, nuanced, and—like many things in nutrition and neuroscience—individualized. While moderate caffeine consumption can offer a variety of cognitive benefits, going overboard may dampen these advantages and introduce cognitive risk factors. Being mindful of your own body's response to caffeine, understanding the timing and dosage, and considering alternative sources of cognitive enhancement can help you navigate this love-hate relationship for your cognitive longevity.

CHAPTER 20: THE MINDFUL SHOPPER: GROCERY SHOPPING FOR BRAIN HEALTH

Introduction

As the saying goes, "You are what you eat." But seldom do we consider that our food choices also sculpt the very core of our identity—our cognition. As you venture into the labyrinth of grocery aisles, remember that each selection is a vote for your future cognitive self. This chapter guides you through a smart and mindful approach to grocery shopping for optimal brain health.

The Grocery List: Planning Before the Plunge

Taking a little time to prepare a list is the first step to avoid the pitfalls of unhealthy, impulsive buying. On this list, prioritize foods that are known to be beneficial for cognitive functions:

- Fruits and vegetables rich in antioxidants like berries, leafy greens, and bell peppers.
- Protein sources like lean meats, fish, and legumes.
- Complex carbs like whole grains, oats, and quinoa.
- Healthy fats including avocados, olive oil, and nuts and seeds.

Seasonal vs. Non-Seasonal Produce

There's something invigorating about consuming fruits and vegetables that are in season. They're not only fresher but also tend to be richer in nutrients. The downside is that seasonal produce can be limited. Non-seasonal items, often imported, can still be good for you but might lack some nutrient potency due to storage and transport times. Balance your choices by mixing seasonal and non-seasonal produce and always aim for variety to maximize the range of nutrients you consume.

Organic, Conventional, and the Middle Path

The organic debate can be polarizing. On one side, organic foods are free from synthetic pesticides and fertilizers, which is a plus. On the flip side, they can be expensive and are not universally better in nutrient content. If you're on a budget, a middle path can be adopted. Consider buying organic versions of produce that you eat regularly and are known to have higher pesticide residues, like strawberries or spinach, while sticking to conventional for items you consume less frequently or those with natural protective layers like oranges or avocados.

Reading Labels: The Quick and the Quirky

Food labels can sometimes read like a puzzle, mixing scientific jargon with marketing gimmicks. Here are some tips:

- Check the serving size and calculate how many servings you are likely to consume.
- Look for high amounts of fiber, vitamins, and minerals and low amounts of sugar and saturated fats.
- Be wary of terms like "all-natural" or "boosts immunity" unless they are backed by reputable certifications.

The Perimeter Strategy: Navigating Aisles

Ever notice how most grocery stores place fresh produce, meat, and dairy products along the perimeter? These foods are less processed and generally healthier. The middle aisles often house processed foods, rich in preservatives and artificial flavors. Following the perimeter strategy during your shopping trip can steer you toward more nutritious options.

Conclusion

Your grocery cart is more than a collection of consumables—it's an investment in your cognitive future. By planning ahead, focusing on seasonality, making educated decisions about organic versus conventional produce, decoding labels efficiently, and adopting effective in-store strategies like the perimeter approach, you can be a more mindful shopper. So, the next time you grab that shopping cart, remember you're not just filling your pantry; you're also nourishing your intellect.

CHAPTER 21: CALORIC RESTRICTION: LESS MIGHT BE MORE

Introduction

The phrase "less is more" might just apply to your daily caloric intake as much as it does to minimalist architecture. Believe it or not, the notion of cutting calories doesn't just shrink your waistline—it may potentially sharpen your wits too.

The Science of Caloric Restriction

Caloric restriction, defined as a reduction in calorie intake without malnutrition, has been shown to extend lifespan in various animal models. The concept is hardly new; in fact, its origins can be traced back to ancient civilizations, where fasting and limited food intake were often a part of cultural or religious practices. Recent studies have evolved this concept from a practice of asceticism to a scientific pursuit. Researchers are increasingly interested in how caloric restriction affects not just longevity but also cognitive health.

In mammals, including humans, caloric restriction has been linked to increased expression of neurotrophic factors like Brain-Derived Neurotrophic Factor (BDNF), a protein essential for maintaining neural plasticity. By improving synaptic connections, BDNF fosters cognitive functions like learning and memory, rendering it a promising avenue for combating age-related cognitive decline.

Caloric Restriction vs. Starvation

Caloric restriction should not be confused with starvation. While both involve a reduction in food intake, starvation is an extreme form of food deprivation that leads to malnutrition, organ failure, and eventually, death. In contrast, caloric restriction aims to reduce caloric intake judiciously, ensuring that essential nutrients are still consumed in adequate amounts.

A good rule of thumb for caloric restriction is a 20-40% reduction in calorie intake compared to what is considered "normal" or "average" for your age, sex, and activity level. Moreover, the focus should be on cutting empty calories—those from foods and beverages high in sugars and fats but low in nutrients—rather than cutting nutrient-rich foods.

A Customized Approach to Caloric Restriction

There is no one-size-fits-all approach to caloric restriction. Factors like age, weight, activity level, and underlying health conditions all come into play. While an athlete in their 20s might safely reduce their daily caloric intake by 500 calories, a sedentary individual in their 60s might only require a 300-calorie cut.

Consulting with healthcare providers like registered dietitians or medical doctors is advisable before embarking on a caloric restriction regimen. They can help customize a plan that not only restricts calories but also ensures that you get the essential nutrients needed for cognitive and overall health.

Risks and Limitations

Caloric restriction isn't a golden ticket to cognitive longevity. Like any dietary intervention, it comes with risks and limitations. For instance, excessive caloric restriction can lead to nutritional deficiencies, loss of muscle mass, and reduced bone density. In certain populations, like those already underweight or with a history of eating disorders, caloric restriction may be contraindicated.

Moreover, the science is still evolving. While animal studies show promising results, long-term studies on the cognitive benefits of caloric restriction in humans are limited. Therefore, it's essential to approach this strategy cautiously, understanding that more research is needed to substantiate its cognitive benefits fully.

Conclusion

Caloric restriction presents an intriguing paradox—the less you eat, the more your brain may benefit. However, it's not a venture to embark upon recklessly. Through informed decisions and medical advice, a measured approach to caloric restriction can be a valuable addition to your cognitive longevity toolkit. It might just prove that when it comes to food and cognition, sometimes less truly is more.

CHAPTER 22: INTERMITTENT FASTING: A TIME TO THINK

Introduction

Time is an enigmatic entity. It marches forward relentlessly, impacting everything in its wake, including our cognitive function. But what if we told you that time—more specifically, timing—could be a potent factor in preserving your mental sharpness? Enter intermittent fasting, an approach to eating that doesn't just ask "what" and "how much," but also "when."

The Science of Intermittent Fasting

Intermittent fasting (IF) is a dietary approach that alternates between periods of fasting and eating. Research suggests that this oscillation influences an array of physiological processes, including metabolism, inflammation, and notably, cognitive function. Cellular repair processes like autophagy are initiated during fasting, which helps in cleaning out damaged cells and reducing oxidative stress. These processes are particularly relevant for brain health, as oxidative stress and inflammation are often associated with cognitive decline.

The Brain's Energy Dilemma

One way intermittent fasting may aid cognitive function is through energy regulation. The brain consumes a staggering amount of energy—around 20% of your daily caloric intake. When you fast, your body shifts from relying on glucose for fuel to breaking down fats into ketones, an alternative energy source that appears to be more efficient for brain cells. The transition to ketone-based metabolism may enhance mental clarity, focus, and even creativity.

Intermittent Fasting and Cognitive Resilience

Cognitive resilience refers to the brain's ability to withstand neurological challenges that could lead to deterioration. Intermittent fasting has been shown to activate stress-response pathways that improve the brain's resilience. In essence, controlled fasting conditions act like a "workout" for your neurons, strengthening them against potential threats like age-related oxidative stress or even neurodegenerative diseases.

Protocols and Practicalities

Intermittent fasting isn't a one-size-fits-all proposition. The 16/8 method, which involves fasting for 16 hours and eating during an 8-hour window, is popular but not universally effective. There's also the 5:2 approach, where you eat normally five days a week and consume only 500-600 calories on two non-consecutive days. Before you delve into intermittent fasting, consult your healthcare provider, especially if you have existing health conditions or are on medications. Moreover, starting slow and giving your body time to adapt can make the transition less jarring.

Cautionary Notes

While the science is promising, it's essential to consider the limitations and potential drawbacks of intermittent fasting. For instance, it may not be suitable for everyone, especially those with certain medical conditions or life stages, like pregnancy. Some people also experience heightened levels of irritability, which may or may not make you the life of the party at social events. And let's not forget: skipping meals might make some cognitive tasks more challenging initially, as your brain adapts to its new fuel regimen.

Conclusion

Intermittent fasting offers a fascinating lens through which to examine the intertwining of nutrition, time, and cognitive function. While not a miracle cure, it does present an intriguing strategy for those seeking to enhance their cognitive longevity. However, it comes with its own set of considerations and potential pitfalls. So, before you let the clock dictate your diet, weigh the evidence, consult experts, and listen to your own body. The key is to find a balanced approach that enriches not just your plate, but your cognitive tapestry.

CHAPTER 23: THE CHEAT DAY DILEMMA: INDULGENCE AND COGNITIVE HEALTH

Introduction

You've stuck diligently to your brain-boosting regimen, but sometimes life throws temptation your way—a birthday cake, a pizza night, or simply the seductive waft of freshly-baked cookies. As you navigate the journey toward cognitive longevity, it's worth considering the role of cheat days. Do these occasional indulgences sabotage your cognitive gains, or could they actually be beneficial?

The Psychology of Cheat Days

The concept of a cheat day implies a break from a monotonous, restrictive diet. While discipline is essential for maintaining a regimen geared toward cognitive health, strict diets can lead to mental fatigue. Cheat days often serve as psychological relief, providing a break that may increase adherence to a diet in the long run. For some people, knowing that they can indulge on a specific day helps them maintain willpower on other days. However, it's essential to understand that "cheating" shouldn't mean gorging on foods with high sugar, salt, and saturated fat levels. Instead, see it as a day to loosen dietary constraints slightly.

Cheat Days and Metabolism

Some proponents of cheat days argue that they serve as a metabolic boost. The idea is that occasional caloric surplus days can stimulate the metabolism and prevent it from slowing down, a common side effect of long-term caloric restriction. However, the science here is inconclusive. There's no definitive proof that cheat days significantly boost metabolism, and doing it too frequently may lead to unhealthy weight gain, offsetting the cognitive benefits achieved through a balanced diet.

Nutritional Consequences

It's easy to nullify a week's worth of nutrient-dense eating with a single day of indulgence. Foods high in sugar, salt, and unhealthy fats can trigger inflammation, potentially affecting the brain's cognitive functions. In particular, these types of foods are associated with insulin resistance, a condition linked to cognitive decline. To minimize the damage, aim for "healthier cheats." Opt for foods that are closer to what you'd normally eat but offer a different flavor profile, such as a spicy vegetable stir-fry instead of a bland quinoa salad.

The Art of Mindful Cheating

If you decide to integrate cheat days into your dietary regimen, aim for a more mindful approach. Savor every bite, eat slowly, and enjoy the aromas and textures. Mindful eating helps you become more aware of satiety cues, making it easier to stop before you overindulge. It also can help you appreciate the contrast between the pleasure of the cheat meal and the wholesome satisfaction of your regular diet, reminding you why you chose the path of cognitive longevity in the first place.

The Social Aspect of Cheat Days

Food is not just about sustenance; it's a social medium. Shared meals strengthen bonds and contribute to emotional well-being, which is also crucial for cognitive health. If your diet is too restrictive, it could isolate you from social gatherings or make you feel awkward during celebratory occasions. Cheat days, if planned well, can coincide with social events, allowing you to partake in communal joy without major cognitive setbacks.

Conclusion

Cheat days are a double-edged sword. On one hand, they can provide psychological relief and might even serve as a metabolic kickstart. On the other, they pose risks of undoing your nutritional gains and triggering inflammation. The key is balance and mindfulness. By making informed choices even on cheat days, you can maintain a path towards cognitive longevity without sacrificing the occasional indulgence. Your brain—and your taste buds—will thank you.

CHAPTER 24: MEAL PREP MINDSET: PLANNING FOR COGNITIVE SUCCESS

Introduction

You've learned about the myriad of foods and eating habits that can help maintain or even boost your cognitive abilities. Now comes the hard part: actually incorporating them into your daily life. This chapter guides you through the process of meal planning and preparation, offering a strategic approach to keep your brain functioning at its peak.

The Cognitive Advantage of Planning Ahead

You may have heard the adage, "Failing to plan is planning to fail." When it comes to diet and cognition, this is especially true. Planning your meals in advance ensures that you'll have all the brain-boosting foods at hand when it's time to eat. Pre-planning minimizes last-minute unhealthy choices, which not only saves your waistline but also your precious neurons. There's also a cognitive boost simply from the act of planning itself; it engages your frontal cortex, the executive center of the brain responsible for complex decision-making and problem-solving.

Building a Weekly Menu

The first step to successful meal prep is building a weekly menu. Start by jotting down recipes that include key ingredients known to enhance cognitive function, such as Omega-3 rich fish, leafy greens high in antioxidants, or whole grains packed with fiber. Having a weekly menu provides structure, making it easier to grocery shop and ultimately saving you time and stress throughout the week. If you have a busy lifestyle, consider preparing dishes in large batches, so they can be easily reheated during hectic times.

Shopping Smart

A well-thought-out shopping list is your best ally when aiming for cognitive longevity through diet. Before you hit the grocery store, make a list of items you'll need for your weekly menu. This not only streamlines your shopping but also minimizes the temptation to indulge in unhealthy options. Place emphasis on the perimeter of the store, where fresh produce, meats, and dairy are located, rather than the aisles filled with processed foods. Remember to include herbs and spices like turmeric and rosemary, which have known cognitive benefits.

Cook in Batches and Portion Control

Batch cooking is the practice of preparing large quantities of meals at one time and storing them for future use. This approach is not only time-saving but can also be a safeguard against unhealthy food choices when you're crunched for time. While cooking in batches, be mindful of portion sizes. Even brain-boosting foods can be detrimental if consumed in large quantities. Portion control is crucial for both weight management and cognitive longevity. Utilize measuring cups or a food scale to ensure you're eating the right amount.

Food Safety and Storage

Nothing ruins a good meal plan faster than food going bad. Invest in quality food storage containers that are airtight to keep your food fresh for longer. Understand the basics of food safety, like cooking meat to the proper temperature and storing perishables correctly. Freezing portions is a good option if you know you won't consume them in a timely manner. Use labels to indicate what's in each container and when it was cooked to avoid any guesswork later.

Conclusion

Meal preparation is more than just a trendy hashtag; it's a key element in maintaining a diet that promotes cognitive longevity. By planning ahead, you can make it easier to incorporate brain-boosting foods into your daily life. Create a weekly menu, shop smartly, cook in batches, and follow food safety guidelines. This systematic approach will not only streamline your eating habits but will also optimize the nutrients beneficial for your brain's health. It's the perfect recipe for cognitive success.

CHAPTER 25: COOKING FOR COGNITION: TECHNIQUES AND RECIPES

Introduction

Eating for cognitive longevity involves more than just choosing the right ingredients; it also requires the proper techniques and recipes to turn these brain-boosting foods into delicious, easy-to-make dishes. In this chapter, let's explore some cooking techniques and recipes that are not just a feast for your taste buds but also for your neurons.

Choosing Cooking Methods Wisely

When it comes to cooking, the method you use can impact the nutrient content and thus, the cognitive benefits of the food. Overcooking vegetables can lead to nutrient loss, while frying can add unwanted trans fats. Opt for steaming, baking, or grilling to retain maximum nutrient value. These cooking methods also utilize less oil, aiding in calorie control.

Cooking Time and Temperature

It's tempting to cook everything on high heat to get it done quicker. However, high heat can destroy some delicate nutrients like vitamin C and some B vitamins. Cooking food at a moderate temperature for a shorter time is often the best approach to maintain its cognitive-boosting potential. When using oils, make sure they have a high smoke point to avoid turning beneficial fats into harmful trans fats.

Spice it Up

Spices like turmeric, ginger, and cinnamon are known for their cognitive benefits. But overcooking spices can lessen their potency. Instead, try adding spices towards the end of the cooking process to preserve their brain-boosting attributes. Similarly, freshly chopped herbs such as basil or parsley can be added as a garnish to not just add flavor but also extra antioxidants.

Incorporating Healthy Fats

We've all heard that Omega-3s are great for the brain. Cooking with oils rich in Omega-3 fatty acids, like flaxseed or walnut oil, can be a good strategy. However, these oils are not suitable for high-heat cooking. They are best used for dressing salads or as a finishing oil. For cooking, extra virgin olive oil or avocado oil, which have moderate smoke points and contain monounsaturated fats, are a better choice.

Recipes to Remember

Here are a couple of easy-to-make, cognitively nutritious recipes that can become regulars in your kitchen repertoire:

Salmon and Quinoa Salad

Ingredients: Cooked quinoa, grilled salmon, baby spinach, walnuts, olive oil, lemon juice, salt, and pepper.

Directions: Toss cooked quinoa, baby spinach, and grilled salmon chunks in a large bowl. Add a handful of walnuts. Make a simple dressing with olive oil, lemon juice, salt, and pepper. Mix well and serve.

<u>Veggie Stir-Fry with Tofu</u>

Ingredients: Tofu, bell peppers, carrots, broccoli, olive oil, garlic, low-sodium soy sauce, and turmeric.

Directions: Sauté minced garlic in olive oil until golden. Add tofu cubes and cook until brown. Throw in the veggies and stir-fry until they soften but still have a crunch. Add a pinch of turmeric and drizzle low-sodium soy sauce for flavor. Serve hot.

Conclusion

Cooking for cognitive longevity isn't just a matter of picking the right foods but also preparing them in ways that maximize their brain-boosting potential. From cooking techniques to time and temperature considerations, all play a part in making your meals both delicious and nutritious. So, tie on that apron and let's get cooking, for the sake of your grey matter!

CHAPTER 26: SUPPLEMENT SAVVY: DO YOU NEED EXTRA HELP?

Introduction

Supplements have long been the subject of both praise and skepticism, acting as the cherry on top for some and a crutch for others. When it comes to cognitive longevity, many people wonder if supplements can offer an added layer of protection. In this chapter, we'll explore the role of supplements in brain health, aiming to separate fact from fiction.

The Hype and the Science

There's no shortage of "magic pills" on the market claiming to boost brainpower. From gingko biloba to fish oil, these supplements often make lofty promises. However, before you part with your hard-earned money, it's essential to understand the scientific basis behind these claims. Clinical trials on these supplements are a mixed bag—some indicate a marginal benefit for specific populations, while others show no effect whatsoever. Make sure you consult the research, and even more importantly, your healthcare provider, before adding a new supplement to your regimen.

Understanding Bioavailability

Bioavailability is the extent and rate at which your body can absorb a substance. Some nutrients in supplement form may not be as bioavailable as those found naturally in food. For example, the antioxidant resveratrol, present in red grapes and red wine, has low bioavailability when taken as a supplement. In contrast, omega-3s in fish oil capsules are highly bioavailable and can serve as an effective alternative to consuming fatty fish. The key takeaway here is that supplements should not be your first option but can sometimes serve as a reasonable alternative.

Is More Better? The Risks of Over-Supplementation

There's a dangerous allure in thinking that if a little is good, then more must be better. The fat-soluble vitamins A, D, E, and K are stored in your body, and excessive intake can lead to toxicity. For instance, overconsumption of vitamin A can lead to dizziness, nausea, and even more severe complications like liver damage. On the flip side, water-soluble vitamins like vitamin C are generally excreted through urine when consumed in excess, making them less risky but not entirely without consequence. Always adhere to recommended dosages and consult your healthcare provider for personalized advice.

The Role of Regulatory Bodies

In many jurisdictions, dietary supplements are not held to the same rigorous testing and quality control standards as pharmaceuticals. This laxity often results in products that may not contain the advertised ingredients or, worse, might contain harmful additives. Consumer protection agencies and various certifications can offer a degree of reliability, but it's always wise to exercise caution and carry out due diligence when selecting a supplement.

Navigating the Supplement Spectrum

If you've done your research and decide that supplementation is right for you, here are a few types commonly associated with cognitive health:

- Omega-3 fatty acids: Known for their anti-inflammatory properties and potential to improve cognitive function.
- Vitamin D: Often recommended for mood regulation and cognitive well-being, especially for those with low sun exposure.
- B Vitamins: These can be particularly useful for people following vegetarian or vegan diets, who might be missing out on B12 found predominantly in animal products.
- Antioxidants like vitamin C and E: Generally recommended for overall health but can also contribute to mental acuity.

It's worth noting that dietary supplements should never serve as a substitute for a balanced diet. Instead, consider them as an auxiliary to fill gaps or provide an extra boost when necessary.

Conclusion

The supplement aisle can be a tantalizing place, offering a plethora of options that promise quick and easy cognitive benefits. However, the best approach is one rooted in evidence and personalized healthcare advice. It's crucial to navigate this landscape cautiously, acknowledging that a balanced diet remains the cornerstone for cognitive longevity. In the end, supplements may offer a supplementary route to brain health, but they're most certainly not a shortcut.

CHAPTER 27: CULINARY CULTURES: WHAT WE CAN LEARN FROM GLOBAL DIETS

Introduction

As you journey through the maze of foods, nutrients, and dietary practices designed to keep your cognition spry, it's worth taking a global perspective. What are other cultures doing right that we can learn from? A food adventure around the world reveals some fascinating trends and habits worth adopting.

The Mediterranean Way: Olive Oil, Fish, and Less Meat

There's a reason the Mediterranean diet consistently ranks high for overall health benefits—it's rich in nutrients beneficial for brain health. Staples like olive oil, nuts, fruits, vegetables, and fish are abundant in omega-3 fatty acids, antioxidants, and other phytonutrients. The Mediterranean populace's penchant for consuming moderate amounts of wine also introduces beneficial antioxidants like resveratrol. So, when thinking about a diet for cognitive longevity, consider adding a Mediterranean flair to your meals.

Japanese Longevity: Seafood and Portion Control

Japan has one of the highest rates of centenarians in the world, and its dietary practices are partly to thank. A traditional Japanese diet is heavy on seafood rich in omega-3s and low in saturated fats and processed foods. The practice of "Hara Hachi Bu," which means eating until you're 80% full, promotes caloric restriction, which, as we've discussed in earlier chapters, can be beneficial for cognitive health. The regular consumption of green tea, high in antioxidants, is another feather in the Japanese diet cap.

The Indian Spice Rack: Turmeric, Cumin, and Ginger

The Indian diet brings an arsenal of spices, each with its unique cognitive benefit. We've talked about curcumin in turmeric; however, other Indian staples like cumin, ginger, and fenugreek also have anti-inflammatory and cognitive-protective properties. Incorporating these spices into your meals not only adds flavor but also boosts your brain's defenses against oxidative stress.

Scandinavian Simplicity: Seasonal and Locally Sourced

The Nordic diet focuses on high-quality, seasonal, and locally sourced foods, reducing the need for processed foods that can deteriorate cognitive function. Berries are a significant component, rich in antioxidants and other brain-beneficial compounds. Fatty fish, whole grains, and root vegetables round out a diet that is simple yet highly effective for maintaining cognitive well-being.

African Roots: Legumes, Tubers, and Leafy Greens

Diets from various African nations often include nutrient-rich foods that are excellent for brain health. Legumes like lentils and chickpeas provide plant-based protein and fiber. Tubers such as sweet potatoes and cassava are complex carbohydrates that provide sustained energy, while leafy greens like collard and mustard greens supply essential vitamins and minerals. Many traditional African diets are low in processed sugars and unhealthy fats, offering a more natural and holistic approach to nutrition.

Conclusion

Sampling global diets is more than a culinary adventure; it offers a treasure trove of practices that promote cognitive longevity. Whether it's the Mediterranean's omega-3-rich fish, Japan's caloric control, India's spice magic, Scandinavia's focus on local and seasonal produce, or Africa's nutrient-packed staples, you can integrate these international wisdoms into your own diet for a sharper mind as you age. So, take your palate on a world tour; your brain will thank you.

CHAPTER 28: BRAIN-FRIENDLY BOOZE? THE ALCOHOL QUESTION

Introduction

Ah, the clinking of glasses, the toast to good health—alcohol has been a social lubricant and culinary companion for centuries. But as we've embarked on a journey toward cognitive longevity, the question arises: How does alcohol fit into the equation? Could a glass of red wine really benefit your brain, or is it merely an elixir of wishful thinking? Let's dig into the neuroscience and nutritional aspects of alcohol's relationship with cognitive health.

The Resveratrol Riddle: Is Red Wine Really Beneficial?

You've probably heard that a glass of red wine a day keeps the doctor away—or something to that effect. This belief primarily stems from the presence of resveratrol, a polyphenol found in red wine, which has been touted for its antioxidant and anti-inflammatory properties. Some studies even suggest that resveratrol could improve brain health and slow down the aging process.

However, it's important to note that the amount of resveratrol you'd have to consume to see significant benefits is far greater than what you can comfortably (or safely) obtain from red wine. Furthermore, excess alcohol consumption can negate any potential benefits by causing oxidative stress and inflammation. So, while it's tempting to raise a toast to resveratrol, moderation is key.

The Good, the Bad, and the Ethanol

Ethanol, the type of alcohol found in beverages, is a double-edged sword. On one hand, moderate drinking—especially of wines and spirits rich in antioxidants—may have some cardiovascular benefits and even improve insulin sensitivity. These factors could, indirectly, support cognitive health.

On the other hand, excessive alcohol consumption is linked to neurodegeneration, brain volume reduction, and cognitive decline. Alcohol disrupts neurotransmitter function and can lead to oxidative stress and inflammation, impairing your brain's ability to repair itself. Moreover, alcohol can interfere with sleep quality, another crucial aspect of cognitive well-being.

The Social Component: A Cognitive Boon or Bane?

For many, alcohol's allure lies in its ability to lighten moods and facilitate social interaction. This social engagement, in turn, is associated with better cognitive health in numerous studies. However, it's a precarious balance; alcohol can also lead to social isolation if misused, not to mention the negative cognitive impacts of alcoholism or binge-drinking behaviors.

The key is responsible enjoyment. Socializing over a glass of wine might bring about positive cognitive effects, provided that the focus remains on quality interactions rather than the quantity of alcohol consumed.

Alcohol and Age: A Shifting Dynamic

As you age, your body's ability to metabolize alcohol changes. The liver becomes less efficient at processing ethanol, and a lifetime's exposure to alcohol can take its toll on liver function and overall cognition. Elderly individuals are often more sensitive to alcohol's effects, including its impact on cognition. Therefore, it's essential to re-evaluate your alcohol consumption habits as you age and consult healthcare professionals for tailored advice.

To Drink or Not to Drink?

If you enjoy a glass of wine or a pint of craft beer, the good news is you don't necessarily have to give it up entirely to maintain cognitive longevity. Moderation and mindful drinking are the mantras. Opt for alcoholic options rich in antioxidants, and always consider the context in which you're consuming alcohol. Is it enhancing your social experience and overall well-being, or is it serving as a crutch that ultimately hampers your cognitive health?

Conclusion

The relationship between alcohol and cognition isn't just complicated; it's a full-blown Shakespearean drama with twists, turns, and ambiguities. While moderate alcohol consumption may offer some benefits, including social engagement, the risks associated with overindulgence are substantial. As with most things in life, and certainly on your quest for cognitive longevity, moderation and context are key. So the next time you find yourself raising a glass, perhaps make it a toast to wisdom and longevity. Cheers.

CHAPTER 29: HORMONES AND HEALTH: EATING FOR HORMONAL BALANCE

Introduction

Hormones are the unseen puppeteers of the body's intricate systems, pulling strings that influence everything from mood to metabolism. And guess what? Diet plays a starring role in this biochemical opera. Welcome to the stage where food meets hormonal balance, and thereby, cognitive function.

Hormones and Cognitive Function: A Tangled Web

Hormones like cortisol, insulin, and the sex hormones estrogen and testosterone have a profound influence on cognitive health. High cortisol levels, often linked to stress, can hamper memory and learning. Elevated insulin levels may impair cognitive function and are associated with the development of neurodegenerative diseases. On the other hand, balanced levels of estrogen and testosterone are essential for optimal neural function, including memory and mood regulation.

A Balanced Plate for a Balanced State

The food you consume can influence the levels of these hormones.

For example, foods rich in omega-3 fatty acids, such as salmon, can help reduce cortisol levels. A balanced diet that includes ample protein can keep insulin levels in check. Consuming soy-based foods like tofu can mimic estrogen effects, potentially beneficial for post-menopausal women at risk of cognitive decline due to low estrogen levels.

Sugar, the Hormonal Wrecking Ball

A high-sugar diet wreaks havoc on your hormonal orchestra, often leading to insulin resistance. Elevated insulin levels can cause a chain reaction of hormonal imbalances, not to mention its adverse effects on cognitive function. It would be prudent to choose complex carbs over simple sugars to ensure a mellifluous hormonal composition conducive to cognitive well-being.

Micronutrients: The Supporting Cast

Vitamins and minerals may not produce hormonal melodies, but they're the stagehands ensuring the show runs smoothly. For example, vitamin D helps in the production of serotonin, a hormone affecting mood and social behavior. A lack of it could lead to cognitive issues. Similarly, magnesium and zinc play roles in the production and regulation of insulin.

Intermittent Fasting and Hormonal Harmony

We've discussed the "what" of eating, but the "when" is just as important. Intermittent fasting, discussed in a previous chapter, can bring about hormonal balance. This eating pattern helps regulate cortisol and insulin levels, enhancing your cognitive potential.

Conclusion

Diet isn't just about calories and nutrients; it's a powerful tool to modulate the symphony of hormones that, in turn, govern your cognitive capacities. By making smart food choices, you can tune your hormonal ensemble to play the sweet melodies of cognitive longevity and well-being.

CHAPTER 30: EATING YOUR EMOTIONS: FOOD AND MOOD

Introduction

You've heard the saying, "You are what you eat." But have you ever considered that what you eat might be influencing how you feel? In this chapter, we'll examine the intricate interplay between food and mood, both of which can be crucial factors in your cognitive longevity.

Nutritional Neuroscience of Mood

There's no denying that the brain is an energy-greedy organ. It requires a steady supply of nutrients to function optimally. Vitamins, minerals, and certain types of fats act as co-factors in the synthesis of neurotransmitters, the brain's messaging molecules responsible for our mood and emotions. For instance, the neurotransmitter serotonin, often termed the "feel-good hormone," is synthesized from the amino acid tryptophan. The availability of tryptophan is influenced by your diet, highlighting how closely your emotional state is tied to what you consume.

Emotional Eating: A Double-Edged Sword

We often resort to food as comfort during emotional distress, reaching for sugary snacks or fatty fast foods. Although such foods may offer momentary relief, they can be detrimental to both your waistline and your brain health. The blood sugar spikes and subsequent crashes that follow the consumption of high-glycemic foods can exacerbate mood swings and irritability. Emotional eating can turn into a vicious cycle, affecting both your cognitive and emotional well-being.

Balanced Meals for Balanced Moods

So what should you eat to stabilize your mood and thereby, support cognitive longevity? A balanced meal containing lean proteins, complex carbohydrates, and healthy fats can do wonders for your emotional state. For instance, omega-3 fatty acids found in fish like salmon have shown potential in reducing symptoms of depression. Additionally, complex carbohydrates like whole grains help in the gradual release of sugar, avoiding the mood swings associated with blood sugar spikes. Micronutrients like magnesium, zinc, and B-vitamins also have roles in mood stabilization.

Microbiota and the Mood Connection

Your gut, often referred to as the 'second brain,' hosts a vast array of microorganisms that significantly impact your mental health. The gut-brain axis is a two-way communication channel, where the health of one can influence the other. Probiotics and prebiotics, beneficial for gut health, can influence the production of neurotransmitters and are being studied for their potential role in alleviating mood disorders like depression and anxiety.

Food as Cognitive Therapy

If you're grappling with chronic stress, anxiety, or mild forms of depression, a strategically planned diet might serve as a complementary treatment method. While not a replacement for professional medical intervention, an optimally planned 'mood diet' may amplify the effects of medication and therapy.

Foods rich in antioxidants like berries and those with anti-inflammatory properties like turmeric can contribute to a more resilient emotional state, thereby supporting cognitive longevity.

Conclusion

The connection between food and mood is intricate yet undeniable. The right nutritional choices can not only improve your emotional well-being but also support your long-term cognitive health. While the focus of the Wisdom Diet is on cognitive longevity, it's empowering to recognize that emotional balance is an integral part of the mental acuity you're striving to achieve. When it comes to diet, it's not just about feeding your intellect; it's also about nourishing your emotional core for a harmonious, cognitive-rich life.

CHAPTER 31: BREAKING BAD HABITS: THE PATH TO BETTER CHOICES

Introduction

After understanding the connection between your diet and cognitive health, it's time to confront the elephant in the room —bad eating habits. We all have them, but the real challenge is breaking free from them to adopt healthier, more brain-friendly routines.

Identifying Bad Habits

The first step in eradicating poor eating habits is acknowledging them. We often underestimate how sneaky these can be. Snacking late at night, eating out of boredom, or resorting to fast food for the sake of convenience—all these are more detrimental to your cognitive health than you might think. These habits can lead to inflammation, poor mental acuity, and long-term cognitive decline.

Behavioral Economics of Eating

Bad habits don't exist in a vacuum; they are the products of an interplay between your environment and psychological triggers.

Stores often place sugary treats at eye level or near the checkout counter because they understand how behavioral economics work. If you're aware of these tricks, you can strategize. For example, make a shopping list and stick to it rigorously. The less you rely on in-the-moment decisions, the more you mitigate the chance of making poor choices.

Replacing With Better Choices

It's not sufficient to merely eliminate bad habits; you have to replace them with good ones. Say you have a penchant for sugary snacks when stressed. Identifying low-glycemic fruits or nuts that you enjoy can provide a satisfying but healthier alternative. Over time, your brain will associate stress-relief with these smarter options, gradually erasing the neural pathways that led you to reach for a doughnut.

Implementing the "Two-Minute Rule"

One of the most intriguing strategies to combat bad habits is the "Two-Minute Rule," a concept rooted in behavioral psychology. It states that if a new habit can be done in two minutes or less, do it immediately. Want to stop yourself from eating a whole bag of chips? Make it a rule to portion out a small bowl and then reseal the bag and put it away. The act of portioning could be your two-minute habit that becomes a stepping stone to larger changes.

Environmental Changes

Don't underestimate the power of your environment in supporting or sabotaging your efforts. Arrange your pantry and fridge so that healthier, brain-boosting options are more accessible than junk food. If you have to work to get to the unhealthy options—by standing on a chair to reach the top shelf or digging behind a pile of vegetables—you'll have that extra moment to consider if it's worth it.

Conclusion

Breaking bad habits is not just an exercise in willpower but a multi-faceted strategy involving awareness, substitution, psychology, and environmental planning. Changing one small habit at a time can set a domino effect into motion, leading to a diet that supports cognitive longevity. Your brain is a masterpiece of evolution, and it deserves nothing less than your best efforts in preserving its functions. After all, the best time to plant a tree was twenty years ago; the second-best time is now. So, take the plunge and make the changes that your future self will thank you for.

CHAPTER 32: THE ORGANIC DEBATE: TO GO ORGANIC OR NOT?

Introduction

Ah, the organic aisle—where produce dons the premium label and the prices make your wallet wince. The question on many a mindful eater's lips: Is going organic really worth it, especially when it comes to enhancing cognitive longevity? In this chapter, we'll slice through the maze of organic versus non-organic and examine whether your brain stands to benefit from this highbrow harvest.

Organic 101: What Does It Even Mean?

First things first, "organic" refers to how agricultural products are grown and processed. Organic farming practices are designed to encourage soil and water conservation, reduce pollution, and utilize fewer synthetic inputs like pesticides, antibiotics, and artificial fertilizers. Sounds dreamy, right? The aim is to cultivate foods that are ostensibly closer to their natural state, though what "natural" means in this context can be up for debate.

Pesticide Predicament: Chemicals and Cognition

One of the most cited reasons for going organic is to avoid pesticide residues on food. While it's true that organic farming employs fewer synthetic pesticides, it's not entirely pesticide-free. Organic farmers often use natural pesticides, which can also be harmful in large quantities. That said, some studies indicate that high levels of certain synthetic pesticides could be linked to cognitive issues, particularly in children. However, the research is still inconclusive regarding the long-term cognitive effects of low-level pesticide exposure in adults.

Nutrient Nuances: Is Organic More Nutritious?

If you've been seduced by the notion that organic foods are nutritionally superior, brace yourself for a reality check. Most comprehensive studies reveal that nutrient content—vitamins, minerals, and antioxidants—doesn't differ significantly between organic and non-organic foods. There are exceptions, of course. For example, some studies suggest that organic dairy products may contain higher levels of Omega-3 fatty acids. But as a general rule of thumb, going organic won't give you a nutrient supercharge capable of morphing you into a cognitive superhero.

Environmental Enlightenment: The Bigger Picture

Organic farming undeniably has a smaller carbon footprint and is often better for soil health and biodiversity. If your concern for cognitive longevity extends to the well-being of the planet (which it should, considering the brain needs a habitable planet to function), organic is a more environmentally friendly choice. However, bear in mind that "organic" doesn't necessarily mean "local" or "sustainable." Transportation and packaging can offset some of the environmental benefits of organic farming.

The Wallet Woe: Affordability and Access

If organic foods were as cheap as their non-organic counterparts, this wouldn't even be a debate. But they aren't. In many regions, organic foods can cost up to 50% more. If you're working within a budget, this can become a significant constraint. There's an argument to be made for prioritizing organic produce when it comes to items you consume in large quantities or those you eat skin and all—like apples or leafy greens. But going full organic might not be financially feasible or cognitively advantageous for everyone.

Conclusion

In the labyrinth of lifestyle choices we navigate for cognitive longevity, going organic seems more like a personal preference rather than a clear-cut cognitive enhancer. While there are valid environmental and potential health reasons to opt for organic, the science has yet to confirm a significant advantage in terms of cognitive longevity. As always, a balanced diet rich in fruits, vegetables, lean proteins, and healthy fats—whether organic or not—remains your best bet for a sharper, more agile mind as you age.

CHAPTER 33: SCREEN TIME SNACKING: THE IMPACT OF DIGITAL DISTRACTION

Introduction

As we navigate the digital age, the boundaries between screen time and mealtime have blurred. Gone are the days of dedicated family dinners; instead, many find themselves munching away in front of a screen. This chapter explores the cognitive implications of this modern behavior and provides insights into making more mindful food choices in an era of perpetual distraction.

The Munching Mind: Why We Snack While Scrolling

A couple of decades ago, the idea of having dinner while watching TV was somewhat frowned upon. Today, the behavior has extended to include snacking while browsing the internet, texting, or working. The question is, why do we find this hybrid activity so compelling?

Neurologically, both eating and screen time release dopamine, the "feel-good" neurotransmitter. The combination amplifies the pleasure, creating a feedback loop that encourages overindulgence in both. It's a classic example of hedonic multitasking, where the brain seeks multiple sources of gratification simultaneously.

Cognitive Costs: The Impact of Distraction on Diet

When your brain is occupied with screen time, the neural networks responsible for making mindful eating decisions are often sidelined. Research suggests that distraction during meals could lead to increased caloric intake. Moreover, the screen's glare and the digital bombardment of information can result in cognitive fatigue, affecting your decision-making abilities. Over time, these distracted eating patterns can contribute to weight gain and cognitive decline, both of which have been shown to adversely affect brain health.

Screen Time and Nutrient Absorption

While it may sound like a stretch, the way your body absorbs nutrients can also be impacted by screen time snacking. Your body requires a certain level of mindful engagement for effective digestion. Eating in front of a screen can impact the release of enzymes needed for digestion. Moreover, stress or excitement from what's on the screen may trigger the release of cortisol, which can further interfere with digestive processes. As a result, even if you're eating brain-boosting foods, you may not be reaping the full cognitive benefits if you're digitally distracted.

Strategies for Mindful Screen Time Snacking

The secret isn't necessarily to eliminate screen time snacking but to engage in it more mindfully. Here are some strategies to consider:

- Set Screen-Free Zones: Designate specific areas of your home for eating and ensure that screens are not part of that landscape.

- Timed Alerts: Use your device to set reminders to stop and consciously think about what you're eating.

- Pre-portion Snacks: Avoid eating directly from a package. Pre-portion your snacks to prevent mindless overeating.

- Choose Cognitive Boosters: If you must snack, opt for foods known to enhance cognitive function, such as berries, nuts, or dark chocolate.

The Digital Plate: Apps for Mindful Eating

Ironically, the very devices that distract us can also aid in mindfulness. There are several apps designed to help you cultivate better eating habits. Apps like "MyFitnessPal" can help you track your caloric intake, while mindfulness apps can guide you through exercises to improve your awareness during meals.

Conclusion

While the allure of double dopamine from screen time and snacking can be strong, it comes at a cognitive cost. By understanding the neurological underpinnings and implications of this behavior, you can take steps to protect your cognitive longevity. Remember, it's not just about eating the right foods; it's also about consuming them in a manner conducive to mental acuity. Your brain deserves the same level of attention that you give to that engrossing article or captivating social media post.

CHAPTER 34: EATING THROUGH THE AGES: ADAPTING YOUR DIET AS YOU AGE

Life, they say, is a journey of change and adaptation. But rarely do we zoom in on the intricacies of this inevitable evolution—especially when it comes to diet and cognitive longevity. As we grow older, our bodies and brains undergo transformations that require a flexible approach to nutritional choices. Let's delve into age-specific strategies to adapt your diet for sustained mental acuity.

The Changing Landscape of Nutrition and Cognition

In your 20s and 30s, it's easy to adopt a cavalier attitude toward diet. A fast metabolism and seemingly boundless energy can often overshadow the long-term ramifications of nutritional choices. However, as you venture into your 40s and beyond, a metabolic slowdown, hormonal changes, and emerging health concerns urge a reevaluation.

The Mighty 20s and 30s

In these decades, focus on building strong cognitive reserves. Your diet should be rich in Omega-3 fatty acids, lean proteins, and a rainbow of fruits and vegetables to foster neural connections. Exercise regularly, and don't skimp on hydration.

The Reflective 40s and 50s

As you transition into midlife, pay attention to maintaining cardiovascular health, crucial for cerebral blood flow. Opt for heart-healthy fats like olive oil and avocados and ramp up on antioxidants like berries and leafy greens to combat oxidative stress.

The Golden 60s and Beyond

Welcome to the years of wisdom. This is the time to counteract age-related muscle loss with adequate protein intake and to focus on calcium and vitamin D for bone health. Brain-wise, lean on foods rich in polyphenols like grapes, cherries, and dark chocolate to support cognitive function.

Cognitive Load and Micronutrient Needs

As we age, our cognitive load—our brain's capacity to process information—changes. Tasks that seemed effortless may now require more mental exertion. With age, the need for certain micronutrients, like B vitamins and vitamin K, increases. These vitamins play vital roles in cognitive health, affecting everything from mood regulation to memory retention.

Tailoring Caloric Intake

An often-overlooked aspect of age-related dietary adaptation is caloric intake. Your energy expenditure generally declines with age, necessitating fewer calories to maintain weight. Yet, your need for nutrients remains constant or may even increase. This calls for "nutrient-dense" foods that deliver the nutritional bang for your caloric buck—think quinoa over white rice, or salmon over processed meats.

Fluid Intelligence and Diet

One cognitive skill that can actually improve with age is "fluid intelligence," the ability to think logically and solve new problems, independent of established knowledge. Research suggests that diets rich in omega-3 fatty acids and antioxidants can further hone this ability.

The Social Context of Eating

Eating is not just a biological necessity; it's a social ritual. As you age, you might find yourself dining alone more often, which can lead to nutritional neglect. Make meals a social event when possible—either virtually or in person. Shared meals not only enrich your social life but also encourage more mindful eating and better nutritional choices.

To conclude, growing older doesn't mean resigning to cognitive decline or settling for sub-optimal nutrition. By adjusting your diet to align with your age-specific needs, you equip your brain with the vital nutrients it requires to function optimally. Remember, it's not just about adding years to your life but adding life to your years—and that includes intellectual vigor. Adapt and thrive, for the best is yet to come.

CHAPTER 35: GENDER MATTERS: TAILORING DIET FOR MEN AND WOMEN

Introduction

Gender-specific nutritional needs aren't just about childbearing or muscle mass; they extend to the realm of cognitive longevity. Both men and women can benefit from understanding how their diet impacts their brain health differently. Let's explore some strategies for each.

Hormonal Variations and Nutritional Needs

The first port of call in gender-specific nutrition is understanding the hormonal landscape. Women experience cyclic hormonal changes and have unique needs during menstruation, pregnancy, and menopause. Consuming foods rich in iron and Vitamin B12 can mitigate cognitive fatigue linked to menstruation. Omega-3 fatty acids, rich in fish and flaxseeds, may help alleviate mood swings.

Men, on the other hand, can experience cognitive effects from testosterone fluctuations. A diet rich in zinc, found in oysters, beef, and lentils, can aid in testosterone production and hence, cognitive clarity.

Satiety and Portion Sizes

Men and women process feelings of fullness differently. This is not merely a caloric difference due to size but a neurochemical one. Leptin, the satiety hormone, behaves differently in both sexes. Research has shown that women may benefit more from fiber-rich foods that offer prolonged satiety and help in weight management, important for hormonal balance. Men, conversely, metabolize fats differently and may not experience quick satiety from fiber alone.

The Calcium Conundrum

Women are often advised to intake more calcium to prevent osteoporosis, especially post-menopause. However, the balance is delicate when it comes to brain health. Some studies suggest excess calcium supplementation could lead to cognitive decline. The idea is to get the right amount of calcium, preferably from dietary sources like leafy greens and dairy, without going overboard.

Aging and Brain Health

Women tend to live longer than men but also experience a higher rate of Alzheimer's disease. The reasons are multi-faceted but estrogen, or the lack thereof after menopause, plays a significant role. Foods rich in phytoestrogens, like soy and flaxseeds, can offer some benefits.

Men, while less prone to Alzheimer's, are more likely to suffer from cognitive issues related to cardiovascular health. Here, a Mediterranean diet rich in fruits, vegetables, and healthy fats can offer preventive benefits.

Special Considerations: Diet and Lifestyle

Both sexes can be vulnerable to the detrimental cognitive effects of poor lifestyle choices, such as smoking or excessive drinking. However, women metabolize alcohol differently and can be more susceptible to its negative cognitive effects. The antioxidant-rich foods that help in detoxification may need to be more prominent in women's diets.

Men, who may be more prone to high-risk behaviors, should consider foods that mitigate stress and enhance focus. Nuts and seeds rich in Vitamin E can offer such cognitive protection.

Conclusion

Gender plays a nuanced role in how diet impacts cognitive longevity. Understanding these differences can empower men and women to make more informed dietary choices. Nutrition isn't one-size-fits-all; your brain will thank you for the customization.

CHAPTER 36: MIND OVER MATTER: THE POWER OF POSITIVE THINKING

Introduction

You've heard it before, "Think positive," but how much weight does this phrase actually carry when it comes to cognitive longevity? As we sail through the discourse on nutrition and neuroscience, let's take a moment to explore another form of nourishment—one that feeds your mind in its quest for mental acuity.

The Placebo Effect in Cognitive Nutrition

We've all heard stories about placebo pills miraculously curing physical ailments, but what about its role in cognitive nutrition? Studies have found that the placebo effect extends to cognitive tasks as well. People who believe they're taking a cognitive enhancer often perform better on tests, even when they're merely ingesting sugar pills. This may not be a green light to chow down on placebos, but it's a stark reminder that belief can set the stage for real physiological change.

Optimism and Cognitive Resilience

Your outlook on life is not just a lens through which you see the world; it also holds potential power over your cognitive abilities. Optimists are shown to handle stress better, which reduces cortisol levels, a hormone known for its detrimental effects on memory and mental acuity. So, while you're chopping up that memory-boosting kale, don't forget to sprinkle a bit of optimism over it.

Self-Efficacy: The Engine of Cognitive Fortitude

Ever met someone who just knows they'll find a way through any challenge? That's self-efficacy at play. This psychological construct is basically your belief in your own ability to execute tasks and achieve goals. Studies have suggested a correlation between high levels of self-efficacy and increased problem-solving abilities, sharper focus, and better memory. As you maneuver through the maze of omega-3s and antioxidants, don't underestimate your inner reservoir of self-efficacy. The road to cognitive longevity might just become a bit less winding.

Mindfulness: The Link to Cognitive Awareness

We've talked about mindful eating, but what about just being mindful—period? Mindfulness is the practice of being fully engaged in the present moment, a mental state where you become an observer of your own thoughts and feelings. The practice has been shown to improve attention span and cognitive flexibility. Mindfulness, when combined with a well-balanced Wisdom Diet, can be the coup de maître in your cognitive longevity strategy.

The Psychological Ripple Effects of Diet Choices

Your choice of brain-boosting foods does more than fuel your neurons; it also influences your mental state. Eating healthy can boost self-esteem and create a virtuous cycle. When you eat well, you feel good about yourself, enhancing your positive outlook and, in turn, further improving your mental faculties. This creates a reinforcing loop of positive dietary habits and better cognitive performance, each boosting the other.

Conclusion

The mind is a complex and enigmatic entity, yet it responds well to simple acts of positivity and belief. As you continue your journey through the labyrinth of nutritional neuroscience, keep in mind that your attitude and mental state serve as valuable co-pilots. They can make your dietary choices more effective and add an extra layer of fortification against cognitive decline. After all, the Wisdom Diet isn't just about what goes into your stomach; it's also about what goes on between your ears.

CHAPTER 37: FAMILY FARE: COGNITIVE NUTRITION FOR ALL AGES

Introduction

Bringing your family along on the journey to cognitive health is not just a compassionate gesture; it's a fundamental step toward a more fulfilling life. When all family members—be they young, old, or in-between—embrace brain-boosting foods, the collective wisdom of the household rises. In this chapter, we explore how the Wisdom Diet can be tailored to meet the needs of family members at various stages of life.

The Early Years: Setting Up for Success

In early childhood, the brain is remarkably plastic, meaning it has a higher ability to change and adapt. For parents of young children, this is the time to introduce a variety of foods rich in essential nutrients like Omega-3s, antioxidants, and proteins. Small swaps like whole grains instead of white bread or fruits instead of sugary snacks can set a lifelong precedent for making healthier choices.

Adolescent Awareness: Brain Food for the Teen Brain

The teenage years are marked by a unique set of challenges: puberty, emotional turbulence, and the onset of adult responsibilities. At this stage, the brain is still in development, particularly the frontal cortex, which is responsible for complex planning, decision-making, and moderating social behavior. Foods rich in Omega-3 fatty acids, such as fish and walnuts, can be particularly beneficial. Additionally, antioxidants from fruits and veggies help in combating oxidative stress, which can affect adolescents who lead a more active, social life.

Adulthood: Maintaining the Cognitive Momentum

Adulthood is often a juggling act between career, family, and personal interests. This busy lifestyle can sometimes make fast food or ready-to-eat meals appear attractive. However, processed foods often contain additives and high levels of salt and sugar, which can be detrimental to cognitive health. Sticking to a diet rich in fruits, vegetables, lean proteins, and whole grains can not only keep you physically fit but mentally agile as well. Keeping a stash of brain-boosting snacks like nuts or fruit slices can make a world of difference during hectic days.

Aging Gracefully: The Golden Years

As people age, the risk for cognitive decline increases. This makes adhering to a brain-healthy diet even more critical. Elderly family members benefit from a diet rich in Omega-3 fatty acids, antioxidants, and a moderate amount of lean protein. Foods like blueberries, salmon, and whole grains are not just heart-healthy; they also have been shown to slow down age-related cognitive decline. Additionally, make sure to keep hydration in check; even mild dehydration can impact mood and cognitive function negatively.

The Family Table: Where Generations Unite

Perhaps the most significant benefit of making cognitive

nutrition a family affair is the strengthening of bonds around the dinner table. Meals can be planned to meet the needs of all age groups. For example, a salmon dinner with a side of quinoa and steamed vegetables offers something for everyone: Omega-3s for brain development in children and adolescents, antioxidants for adults juggling daily stresses, and essential nutrients for the elderly. Add a dessert of mixed berries, and you've got a meal that's a cognitive powerhouse.

Conclusion

While individual needs may vary with age, the goal remains constant: boosting cognitive health through nutrition. By adapting the Wisdom Diet to each family member's unique requirements, you're not just improving individual well-being; you're elevating the health of your entire household. So, gather around the table—it's time to eat wisely and think wisely, together.

CHAPTER 38: CULINARY CREATIVITY: MAKING HEALTHY EATING ENJOYABLE

Introduction

Let's face it; the prospect of a lifetime of brown rice, steamed vegetables, and lean proteins can seem, well, a bit bland. However, eating for cognitive longevity doesn't have to be a dreary, monotonous affair. With a little ingenuity in the kitchen, you can make your meals as vibrant and diverse as a tropical coral reef, while still catering to the nutritional needs of your brain.

Spice it Up

The role of spices in brain health has been covered in previous chapters, specifically highlighting the importance of curcumin, found in turmeric. But spices do more than enhance cognitive function; they also add a burst of flavor to your meals. Cinnamon, for instance, pairs well with both sweet and savory dishes, and it has been linked to improved insulin sensitivity. Fresh herbs like rosemary, thyme, and basil not only add a fragrant aroma to your dishes but also pack a phytonutrient punch. Get creative by blending spices and herbs to create your own unique seasoning mixes.

The Color Spectrum

Visual appeal can significantly influence your enjoyment of a meal. Studies have indicated that we are more likely to eat, and even enjoy, colorful meals compared to monochrome ones. In fact, the range of colors in vegetables and fruits often indicates a variety of essential nutrients. Reds and purples in berries, oranges and yellows in citrus fruits, and greens in leafy vegetables—all these contribute to a variety of nutritional benefits including antioxidants, vitamins, and fiber. Remember, your plate should resemble an artist's palette, not a blank canvas.

Reimagine Your Favorites

Eating brain-healthy foods doesn't mean giving up on your favorite dishes; it's about adapting them. Love spaghetti? Try spiralized zucchini instead of traditional pasta. Are burgers your weakness? Opt for a grilled portobello mushroom cap instead of a beef patty, or make a ground turkey patty seasoned with brain-friendly spices. Craving pizza? Use a cauliflower crust and top it with nutrient-rich vegetables and a dash of olive oil. The key is to swap out less healthy ingredients for options that are rich in nutrients beneficial for cognitive longevity.

Culinary Techniques: Beyond Boiling

Cooking methods can alter the nutritional profile of your food. For instance, boiling vegetables might leach out some water-soluble nutrients. Why not try steaming, grilling, or roasting instead? Slow cooking is another excellent way to preserve nutrients while deepening flavors. Consider using a sous-vide for proteins to maintain their moisture and nutrient content. Even the oils you use for cooking matter; opt for those rich in omega-3s and antioxidants, like extra virgin olive oil or avocado oil. A slight change in cooking technique can transform a mundane dish into a culinary masterpiece.

Reinventing Snacks

Even snacking can be both enjoyable and brain-healthy. Replace chips with air-popped popcorn seasoned with nutritional yeast for a cheesy flavor without the dairy. Make your own trail mix with nuts, seeds, and a sprinkle of dark chocolate chips. Or go for fruit slices dipped in a small amount of almond butter. These small changes make snacking a fun experience without compromising on cognitive health.

Conclusion

Eating for cognitive longevity isn't about sentencing yourself to a lifetime of bland, uninteresting foods. With a sprinkle of culinary creativity, you can enjoy a diet that's as delicious as it is beneficial for your brain. So, put on that apron and let the kitchen become your playground, keeping your meals—and your mind—as vibrant as ever.

CHAPTER 39: TRAVELER'S MIND: EATING WISELY ON THE GO

As they say, the world is a book, and those who do not travel read only one page. But what happens when the globe-trotter in you worries about maintaining cognitive acuity while navigating foreign menus or airport snack bars? In this chapter, we'll explore how you can maintain the Wisdom Diet while you're far from home, ensuring that you keep your brain as sharp as your sense of adventure.

The Prepared Voyager: Packing Brain-Boosting Snacks

Before embarking on your journey, it's wise to pack a small arsenal of brain-boosting snacks. Trail mixes with almonds, walnuts, and dark chocolate bits offer a scrumptious but effective combination of Omega-3s and antioxidants. Consider packing portable fruits like apples or oranges, which can add a splash of brain-friendly vitamin C to your travel itinerary. These handy snacks can become your go-to alternatives when confronted with fast-food outlets or less-than-ideal eating choices.

Reading Foreign Menus: A Brain Workout

A complex foreign menu can feel like a cognitive test, but with a little preparation, you can navigate it wisely. Research the dietary staples of your destination beforehand, so you know what items are likely to fit the Wisdom Diet. Words like "grilled," "steamed," or "baked" usually indicate healthier options, whereas "fried" or "cream" should raise red flags. This is not just about making wise choices; it's also a mental exercise in itself, akin to a real-world puzzle your brain has to solve.

Airports and Pit Stops: The Gauntlet of Temptation

The airport can be a minefield of sugary traps and high-carb pitfalls. Coffee shops tempting you with sugary lattes and pastries can test your resolve. Opt instead for a green tea and a piece of whole-grain toast if available. Many airports also have salad bars or offer pre-packaged salads. Just be cautious with the dressings; opt for olive oil or a squeeze of lemon to keep the Omega-3 to Omega-6 ratio in check.

Street Food and Local Delicacies: An Adventure in Moderation

Street food can be one of the most memorable aspects of travel. While sampling local delicacies is part of the cultural experience, it should also be approached with a grain of proverbial salt. Fried or sugary treats can be enjoyed occasionally, but don't make them a staple of your travel diet. Remember, you're not just a traveler in space; you're also a traveler in time, journeying into your older years. Make choices that your future self will thank you for.

Travel-Friendly Apps and Tools: Digital Aides for Smart Eating

In this digital age, your smartphone can be a powerful ally in maintaining cognitive longevity. Apps like MyFitnessPal can help you track your calorie and nutrient intake, even when you're dealing with foreign cuisine. Translation apps can also assist in deciphering menus, while Yelp or TripAdvisor can offer insights into the healthier dining options available in your area.

Summary

Staying true to the Wisdom Diet while traveling doesn't mean you have to sacrifice the culinary adventure that comes with exploring new places. It's entirely possible to enjoy what the world has to offer in food while making choices that align with cognitive longevity. With some forethought, wise use of technology, and a commitment to balance and moderation, you can ensure that your travel experiences enrich not just your soul, but also your brain.

CHAPTER 40: CONCLUSION: THE ROAD AHEAD

As we bring our culinary and cognitive journey to a close, it's clear that the fork and knife you wield at the dinner table are also tools for sculpting the architecture of your mind. The strategies and insights offered through the course of this book aim not just to enhance the taste of your meals but to nourish the very substrate of your thoughts, emotions, and memories.

Integrating The Wisdom Diet into Daily Life

Adapting your diet for cognitive longevity isn't a one-time event; it's a lifestyle commitment. Keeping the tenets of The Wisdom Diet at the forefront of your decision-making ensures that you continually reap its benefits. From scrutinizing nutritional labels to experimenting with antioxidant-rich recipes, these practices must become as automatic as brushing your teeth.

Revisiting Your Cognitive Baseline

Periodic self-assessment is an important part of this dietary journey. Utilize memory tests, mood evaluations, and even medical check-ups to measure the effectiveness of your dietary changes. This not only provides motivation but helps you tweak your approach to better align with your cognitive goals.

Lifelong Learning and Adaptation

New research in nutritional neuroscience is emerging all the time. Stay abreast of current studies and be prepared to fine-tune your dietary strategy as new information becomes available. Just as you wouldn't use an outdated map to navigate a modern city, don't rely on obsolete information when the landscape of nutritional science is constantly evolving.

Broadening Your Culinary Horizons

The Wisdom Diet isn't just about what you should or shouldn't eat; it's about enjoying the process of discovery. Continue to experiment with spices from far-off lands, learn recipes that stimulate more than just your taste buds, and perhaps even enroll in a cooking class focused on brain-healthy foods. After all, cognitive longevity is not merely the absence of decline; it's the continual enrichment of your mental landscape.

Passing It On: The Wisdom Diet as a Family Legacy

Your pursuit of cognitive longevity shouldn't be a solitary expedition. Involve your family, particularly if you have young children or elderly parents, in this enlightening journey. The family table is where many lifelong habits, both good and bad, take root. Let your dinner table be a breeding ground for cognitive vitality that spans generations.

The Wisdom Diet isn't a magic pill, nor is it a panacea that promises immortality. What it offers is a scientifically grounded, nutritionally sound pathway to a future where your cognitive faculties continue to serve you well. Even as the calendar pages turn, your ability to think clearly, remember vividly, and engage meaningfully doesn't have to fade into the twilight of your years. So, go ahead—relish that omega-3 rich salmon, indulge in that blueberry-packed smoothie, and cherish that cup of antioxidant-rich green tea. Here's to not just more years in your life, but more life in your years.

THE END

Printed in Great Britain
by Amazon